Orthostatic Hypotension in Older Adults

Ahmet Turan Isik • Pinar Soysal

Editors

Orthostatic Hypotension in Older Adults

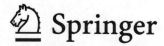 Springer

Editors
Ahmet Turan Isik
Department of Geriatric Medicine, Faculty
of Medicine
Dokuz Eylul University
Izmir
Turkey

Pinar Soysal
Department of Geriatric Medicine, Faculty
of Medicine
Bezmialem Vakif University
Istanbul
Turkey

ISBN 978-3-030-62495-8   ISBN 978-3-030-62493-4   (eBook)
https://doi.org/10.1007/978-3-030-62493-4

This Springer imprint is published by the registered company Springer Nature Switzerland AG
The registered company address is: Gewerbestrasse 11, 6330 Cham, Switzerland

Preface

Orthostatic hypotension (OH) is defined as a certain amount of decrease in blood pressure in the first 3 min of transition from the supine position to the upright position. The prevalence, which increases with advancing age, varies between 20% and 30% in patients over 65 years of age. Besides, it is a medical problem resulting from the deterioration of the adaptation ability of the body with advancing age.

OH is associated with various adverse health outcomes, such as coronary heart disease, congestive heart failure, stroke, falls, dementia, and all-cause mortality. On the other hand, a range of comorbidities, which are common in older adults, and several medications may also play a role in the development of OH.

With multiple etiologies, OH is a significant cause of morbidity and mortality in the elderly. Therefore, it may be referred to as a geriatric syndrome that affects daily life activities and impairs quality of life. For this reason, in order not to overlook OH in the elderly, postural blood pressure changes should be evaluated routinely, as an essential part of the comprehensive geriatric assessment.

We decided to prepare the book *Orthostatic Hypotension in Older Adults* in order to examine OH in all aspects, which is such an important health problem for geriatric patients and to discuss the most rational approaches in this regard. It is our greatest happiness that the book will complement an important deficiency in geriatric practice.

We would like to thank all the scientists for their valuable contributions to the creation of the book by preparing the relevant chapters in the light of their knowledge and experience.

We wish that the book *Orthostatic Hypotension in Older Adults* will be beneficial to scientists and health professionals related to the subject.

Izmir, Turkey   Ahmet Turan Isik
Istanbul, Turkey   Pinar Soysal

Contents

Mechanisms of Orthostatic Tolerance and Age-Related Changes in Orthostatic Challenge

Fatma Sena Dost Gunay and Ozge Dokuzlar

1.1 Introduction

Orthostatic tolerance is a term that defines the ability to prevent hypotension during gravity stress. [1]. First, maintaining postural balance and homeostasis requires the integration of sensory information through proprioception, visual and vestibular pathways [2]. Visual and vestibular stimulation is confounded by proprioceptive input from stretched legs and joint and this integration is important for postural stability, blood pressure, and muscle activity [3]. The regulation of blood pressure (BP) depends on the proper function of the muscle pump, cardiac, renal, neural (parasympathetic and sympathetic nervous systems, baroreflex), and endocrine systems [4, 5].

1.2 Mechanisms of Orthostatic Tolerance

1.2.1 Cardiac Mechanism

In the upright position due to the gravity, 500–700 mL of blood translocates from the upper body to the lower limbs and splanchnic circulation and approximately 10% of the intravascular plasma shifts towards the extravascular space [6, 7]. Venous return and ventricular filling decrease because of that mechanism. Reduction of ventricular filling results in decreased cardiac output and BP. Ventricular filling pressure (end-diastolic volume) indicates the left ventricular end-diastolic diameter. Changes in leftventricular end-diastolic diameter alter the ability of the leftventricular force and thereby stroke volume (SV) [8]. This situation is based on Frank-Starling relationship. Increased end-diastolic volume causes increased sarcomere

F. S. Dost Gunay · O. Dokuzlar (✉)
Department of Geriatric Medicine, Dokuz Eylul University, Faculty of Medicine, Izmir, Turkey

© Springer Nature Switzerland AG 2021
A. T. Isik, P. Soysal (eds.), *Orthostatic Hypotension in Older Adults*, https://doi.org/10.1007/978-3-030-62493-4_1

length and powerful contraction of the left ventricle. There is a relationship between stroke volume and sarcomere length to a degree [9]. In the upright position due to reduced venous return, end-diastolic volume decreases. Decreased end-diastolic volume and sarcomere length causes diminished stroke volume. The normal heart maintains its output by several mechanisms, such as Frank-Starling relationship, increasing heart rate, peak force, and elevation of afterload [10]. There is a two-part increase in BP, one of which is splanchnic vasoconstriction and the other is increased heart rate [11]. Increased heart rate is due to increased adrenaline secretion [12].

1.2.2 Parasympathetic and Sympathetic Nervous Systems (Baroreflex)

Baroreceptor stimuli cause baroreflex (BR). Baroreceptors are sensitive to pressure and strain and are located in the heart's auricles, heart fat pads, vena cava, aortic arch, and carotid sinus wall. As a result of baroreceptor stimulation, the parasympathetic nervous system is activated, while the sympathetic nervous system is inactivated [13]. In the upright position, the ventricular wall tension decreases as a result of the decrease in the ventricular volume. In this case, BR is a typical compensatory reflex mechanism to a reduction in stroke volume, which is manifested by increased heart rate, cardiac contractility, and peripheral vascular resistance [3]. Cardiac BR is responsible for the heart rate and sympathetic BR for BP [14]. Vagal withdrawal and activation of the sympathetic nervous system are the basis of the baroreflex. This mechanism helps restore cardiac output and BP for a few beats [15]. After this short-term compensation, the muscle pump mechanism is activated to maintain blood pressure.

1.2.3 Muscle Pump Reflex

During upright position, skeletal muscles (especially lower extremity muscles) help to maintain venous return by compressing the veins, which is called a skeletal muscle pump mechanism. The muscle pump mechanism is very effective, so a single muscle contraction may direct more than 40% of the intramuscular blood volume to the venous return [16]. Even while standing silently, the lower limb muscle tension and this rhythmic activity act to maintain balance and reduce the amount of blood redistributed due to gravity [17]. In the upright position, muscle pump mechanism after short-term cardiac compensation is the most important mechanism for the maintenance of BP.

1.2.4 Renal and Endocrine Systems

When blood pressure drops below normal, decreased blood pressure directly affects the kidneys, increasing water and salt retention. A decrease in arterial pressure causes an increase in the secretion of aldosterone.

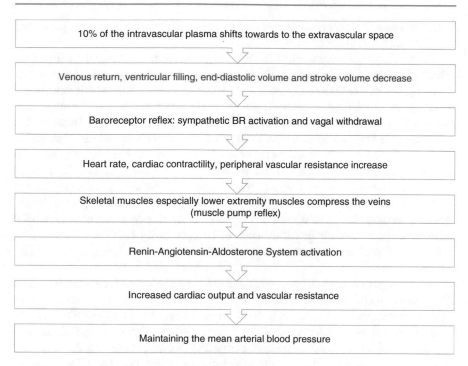

Fig. 1.1 Response mechanism in the uprightposition

First of all, arterial pressure drop increases renin release from juxtaglomerular cells. Renin increases the secretion of angiotensin, which stimulates aldosterone secretion from the adrenal gland. A decrease in blood pressure also directly causes aldosterone secretion which increases water and salt retention from renal tubules. Increased salt absorption increases water retention by increasing antidiuretic hormone (ADH), leading to vasoconstriction with the action of ADH. The increase in body fluid volume, in turn, returns the arterial pressure toward normal [18] (Fig. 1.1).

1.3   Age-Related Changes in Orthostatic Challenge

Aging brings about many physiological differences in the body that cause both structural and functional changes. Therefore, with advancing age, it is difficult to provide the homeostatic balance against stress factors [19]. Age-related decreases are observed in orthostatic tolerance mechanisms as in many other systems [20]. Vision and vestibular systems are of great importance in the upright position. With aging, the deterioration of visual functions affects perception and the activities of older adults [21]. Vestibulosympathetic reflex also deteriorates in older adults, and maintaining arterial blood pressure in the upright position becomes more difficult [22]. All three phases of the orthostatic challenge: [1] an initial heart rate rise and blood pressure drop, [2] an early phase of stabilization, and [3] a phase of prolonged stabilization are influenced by aging [23].

There is a progressive decline in cardiovagal baroreflex sensitivity with aging, which leads to an inadequate heart rate response to a change in blood pressure. Although all of the underlying mechanisms are not clear, arterial stiffness in the baroreceptor-containing segments (such as carotid artery and aorta), decreased cardiac cholinergic response, and oxidative stress are some of the causes. In contrast to this decline in vagal baroreflex sensitivity, no age-related changes were observed in the baroreflex-mediated sympathetic outflow [24]. However, in older age, the number of pacemakers in the sinoatrial node decreases. Also, a decrease in beta-adrenoreceptor-mediated response to norepinephrine is observed. This may be due to beta-adrenoreceptor downregulation caused by high norepinephrine levels. Another cardiac change is decreased diastolic filling due to a decrease in cardiac compliance and preload. In the absence of compensatory cardioacceleration, the reduction of preload may cause a remarkable reduction in cardiac output [20, 25, 26].

In an upright position, a concurrent increase in peripheral vascular resistance is important to maintain blood pressure regulation additively to baroreflex-mediated cardiac compensation. However, another impaired orthostasis mechanism in older adults is the reduced vasoconstrictor response to alpha 1-adrenergic stimulation and the absence of an expected increase in peripheral vascular resistance. Although the responsible mechanisms are not clear, a decrease in vascular compliance due to atherosclerosis, deterioration in norepinephrine re-uptake and release, and a decrease in the number of alpha receptors in vascular smooth muscle are the possible causes [27] (Fig. 1.2).

Aging impairs not only autonomic regulation but also skeletal muscle function. While standing, in addition to the autonomic control of blood pressure, the lower leg muscles play an important role in maintaining blood pressure by pumping the pooled venous blood back to the heart. Also, according to known mechanical muscle pump knowledge to push venous blood back into the heart, activation of leg muscles has been shown to depend on blood pressure fluctuations, i.e.,

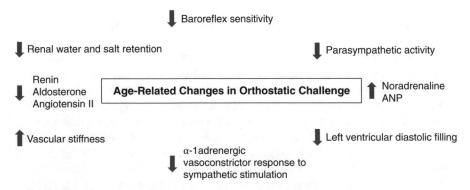

Fig. 1.2 Mechanisms of age-related changes in orthostatic challenge

muscle-pump baroreflex. Therefore, the postural system (leg muscle activation) also contributes to orthostasis while standing. However, studies have found that in older adults, muscle pump baroreflexes, especially in lateral gastrocnemius and soleus muscles, are lower than younger ones. These findings can be important to improve specific exercise or training strategies to restrain aging-related impairment in muscle-pump baroreflexes [28]. Neuroendocrine changes are the other compensator mechanisms for hemodynamic homeostasis, especially in long-term maintenance. However, it is known that the activity of RAAS decreases with advancing age. Both absolute levels and responses to stimulation of plasma renin and angiotensin II concentrations decrease. Some reasons for the decrease are nephrosclerosis, reduced renal mass, and impaired juxtaglomerular cell function in the aging kidney. On the other hand, a strong renin and aldosterone secretion inhibitor ANP plasma levels increase with advancing age. This is another cause of RAAS inhibition [29]. In addition, the feeling of thirst decreases with age, and the aging kidney reduces the ability to concentrate urine; therefore, older adults become inclined to dehydration. Of course, dehydration is an important risk factor for orthostatic intolerance [20, 29].

Orthostatic hypotension (OH) is common in older adults due to the inadequacy of the mentioned mechanism, and OH is closely related to mortality and morbidity [30].

1.4   Conclusion

Aging is a risk factor for orthostatic intolerance with its physiological changes. Therefore, we should avoid additional interventions and treatments that could adversely affect homeostatic mechanisms maintained at the border to protect older adults from orthostatic hypotension.

References

1. Claydon VE, Norcliffe LJ, Moore JP, Rivera-Ch M, Leon-Velarde F, Appenzeller O, et al. Orthostatic tolerance and blood volumes in Andean high altitude dwellers. Exp Physiol. 2004;89(5):565–71.
2. Dichgans J, Diener HC. The contribution of vestibulo-spinal mechanisms to the maintenance of human upright posture. Acta Otolaryngol. 1989;107(5–6):338–45.
3. Garg A, Xu D, Laurin A, Blaber AP. Physiological interdependence of the cardiovascular and postural control systems under orthostatic stress. Am J Physiol Heart Circ Physiol. 2014;307(2):259–64.
4. Chopra S, Baby C, Jacob JJ. Neuro-endocrine regulation of blood pressure. Indian J Endocrinol Metab. 2011;15(Suppl4):S281–8.
5. Joseph A, Wanono R, Flamant M, Vidal-Petiot E. Orthostatic hypotension: a review. Nephrol Ther. 2017;13:S55–67.
6. Mathias CJ. To stand on one's own legs. Clin Med. 2002;2(3):237–45.
7. Jacob G, Ertl AC, Shannon JR, Furlan R, Robertson RM, Robertson D. Effect of standing on neurohumoral responses and plasma volume in healthy subjects. J Appl Physiol. 1998;84(3):914–21.

8. Sarnoff SJ, Mitchell JH. The regulation of the performance of the heart. Am J Med. 1961;30(5):747–71.
9. Braunwald E. Pathophysiology of heart failure. In: Heart Disease. 4th ed. Philadelphia; WB Saunders; 1992. p. 393.
10. Sequeira V, van der Velden J. Historical perspective on heart function : the frank – Starling law. Biophys Rev. 2015;7(4):421–47.
11. Lehndorff A. Über die ursachen der typischen schwankungen des allgemeinen blutdruckes bei reizung der vasomotoren. Archiv für Physiol. 1908:362–91.
12. Elliott TR. The control of the suprarenal glands by the splanchnic nerves. J Physiol. 1912;44(5–6):374–409.
13. Groenland EH, Spiering W. Baroreflex amplification and carotid body modulation for the treatment of resistant hypertension. Curr Hypertens Rep. 2020;22(4):27.
14. Porta A, Marchi A, Bari V, De Maria B, Esler M, Lambert E, et al. Assessing the strength of cardiac and sympathetic baroreflex controls via transfer entropy during orthostatic challenge. Philos Trans R Soc A Math Phys Eng Sci. 2017;375(2096):20160290.
15. Verma AK, Garg A, Xu D, Bruner M, Fazel-Rezai R, Blaber AP, et al. Skeletal muscle pump drives control of cardiovascular and postural systems. Sci Rep. 2017;7:1–8.
16. Stewart JM, Medow MS, Montgomery LD, McLeod K. Decreased skeletal muscle pump activity in patients with postural tachycardia syndrome and low peripheral blood flow. Am J Physiol Circ Physiol. 2004;286(3):H1216–22.
17. Masterson MM, Morgan AL, Cipriani D. The role of lower leg muscle activity in blood pressure maintenance of older adults. Clin Kinesiol. 2006;60:8–17.
18. Guyton AC, Coleman TG, Cowley AW, Scheel KW, Manning RD, Norman RA. Arterial pressure regulation. Overriding dominance of the kidneys in long-term regulation and in hypertension. Am J Med. 1972;52(5):584–94.
19. Navaratnarajah A, Jackson SHD. The physiology of ageing. Medicine. 2017;45(1):6–10.
20. Gupta V, Lipsitz LA. Orthostatic hypotension in the elderly: diagnosis and treatment. Am J Med. 2007;120(10):841–7.
21. Pastalan LA. The simulation of age-related sensory losses: a new approach to the study of environmental barriers. J Vis Impair Blind. 1974;68(8):356–62.
22. Monahan KD, Ray CA. Vestibulosympathetic reflex during orthostatic challenge in aging humans. Am J Physiology Regul Integr Comp Physiol. 2002;283(5):R1027–32.
23. Kenny RA, Cunnigham C. Synco Spe. In: Halter JB, Ouslander JG, Studenski S, High KP, Asthana S, Ritchie CS, Supiano MA, editors. Hazzard's geriatric medicine and gerontology 7th edition. New York: McGraw-Hill Education; 2017. p. 949–68.
24. Monahan KD. Effect of aging on baroreflex function in humans. Am J Physiol Regul Integr Comp Physiol. 2007;293(1):R3–12.
25. Hajjar I. Postural blood pressure changes and orthostatic hypotension in the elderly patient: impact of antihypertensive medications. Drugs Aging. 2005;22(1):55–68.
26. Rehman HU, Masson EA. Neuroendocrinology of ageing. Age Ageing. 2001;30(4):279–87.
27. Sugiyama Y, Matsukawa T, Shamsuzzaman AS, Okada H, Watanabe T, Mano T. Delayed and diminished presser response to muscle sympathetic nerve activity in the elderly. J Appl Physiol. 1996;80(3):869–75.
28. Verma AK, Xu D, Garg A, Blaber AP, Tavakolian K. Effect of aging on muscle-pump Baroreflex of individual leg muscles during standing. Front Physiol. 2019;10:845.
29. Phillips PA, Hodsman GP, Johnston CI. Neuroendocrine mechanisms and cardiovascular homeostasis in the elderly. Cardiovasc Drug Ther. 1991;4:1209–13.
30. Soysal P, Yay A, Isik AT. Does vitamin D deficiency increase orthostatic hypotension risk in the elderly patients? Arch Gerontol Geriatr. 2014;59(1):74–7.

Orthostatic Hypotension: A New Geriatric Syndrome

2

Pinar Soysal and Ahmet Turan Isik

The life expectancy and world population have started to increase significantly in parallel with the developments in science, technology, and health since the mid-nineteenth century and led to the emergence of geriatrics discipline in the early twentieth century. In addition, due to age-related changes that occur with advancing age, general Hippocratic medicine has been replaced by syndromal medicine and the concept of "geriatric syndromes" has emerged [1]. Unlike the concept of "disease," geriatric syndromes occur due to multifactorial causes.So far, dementia, delirium, depression, incontinence, falls, polypharmacy, malnutrition, pressure sores, sarcopenia, and frailty have been accepted as geriatric syndrome [1]. In a study involving 2816 older patients, it was found that prevalence was 54.5% for polypharmacy, 47.6% for urinary incontinence, 9.6% for malnutrition, 35.1% for depression, 21.6% for dementia, 33.6% for falls, 31.7% for sarcopenia, 28.3% for frailty, and 1.1% for pressure ulcers. In the same study, all geriatric syndromes, except for depression and pressure ulcers, were determined to be significantly more common with advancing age [1].While the rate of having four or more syndromes in the same person was 27.1%, 12% had no geriatric syndrome, 22.9% had one syndrome, and 21% had two syndromes. In particular, the frequency of having three or more syndromes in the same age group at ≥80 years was calculated as 68.8% [1].

Common Features of Geriatric Syndromes
1. The frequency increases with age.
2. Multiple pathological processes accompany the event.

P. Soysal (✉)
Department of Geriatric Medicine, Faculty of Medicine, Bezmialem Vakif University, Istanbul, Turkey
e-mail: psoysal@bezmialem.edu.tr

A. T. Isik
Department of Geriatric Medicine, Faculty of Medicine, Dokuz Eylul University, Izmir, Turkey

© Springer Nature Switzerland AG 2021
A. T. Isik, P. Soysal (eds.), *Orthostatic Hypotension in Older Adults*,
https://doi.org/10.1007/978-3-030-62493-4_2

3. Many causes play a role in etiology and are easily complicated.
4. Multiple organs are affected.
5. The clinic can be quite faint and atypical presentation is common.

Considering the common features of geriatric syndromes, the question arises whether orthostatic hypotension (OH) can also be a geriatric syndrome.

2.1   Is OH a Geriatric Syndrome?

1. Does the frequency increase with age?

In a review that examined the age-related increase of OH prevalence and the results of two separate epidemiological studies, it was stated that changes such as increase in age and vascular stiffness associated with age, decrease in barore-flex sensitivity, and decrease in beta adrenoreceptor response may increase OH development [2].The first of these studies was conducted by Rose et al. involving 12,433 people between the ages of 45 and 65, and it was shown that the frequency of OH increased compared to the five-year age ranges and after 6 years of follow-ups, it was found that cardiovascular mortality was higher in those with OH. In the second study by Rutan et al., it was found that in 5201 people over 65 years of age, OH increased with age (that it has increased exponentially especially after the age of 80) and the presence of OH was associated with the development of cardiovascular events when followed for 3 years [2–4]. There are many similar study results in the literature.

2. Do more than one pathological process accompany the event?

Numerous factors play a role in the development of OH, just like other geri-atric syndromes: [2, 5].

- In arteries and veins, stiffness and curvature increase, and baroreceptor sensi-tivity decreases.
- Cardiac hypertrophy due to old age and diastolic filling defect due to hyper-tension occur.
- Renal sodium retention decreases.
- Renin–angiotensin–aldosterone level decreases.
- Sensitivity to hormones such as arginine and vasopressin decreases.
- The maximum increase in heart rate expected during hypotensive maneuvers decreases with age. (In other parts of the book, the pathogenesis of OH is explained in more detail.)

3. Why are multiple factors involved in etiology and are they easily complicated?

In addition to the numerous pathophysiological changes that occur with aging, some other factors may increase the severity of OH or cause the develop-ment of OH in someone who does not have OH before. These situations are generally evaluated under two headings as acute and chronic. Acute OH causes usually develop in a short time and are symptomatic, of which adrenal insuffi-ciency, myocardial ischemia, drug applications, sepsis, and dehydration are examples. Chronic OH causes take long time to develop and are generally asymptomatic at the beginning. It can also occur as a result of various physiological or pathological processes. Physiological causes include the age-related changes mentioned above in the regulation of blood pressure. Pathological causes may be autonomic deficiencies secondary to central or peripheral nervous system diseases [6].

Drugs in etiology are also important because OH is a common cause and drug-induced OH is easier to prevent and correct. In the study conducted by Poon et al., they found that the prevalence of OH was 35%, 58%, 60%, and 65% among those who never used drugs, who used 1 drug, who used 2 drugs, and who used 3 or more drugs, respectively [7].It has been highlighted in previous studies that hypnotic and antidepressant medication use and falls have been associated with elderly individuals who should be particularly evaluated in terms of drug-related OH [8].Soysal P. et al. evaluated 407 geriatric outpatients with the head-up tilt table test and demonstrated thatthe mean age, recurrent falls, presence of dementia and Parkinson's disease, number of drugs, alpha-blocker and anti-dementia drug use, and fasting blood glucose levels were significantly higher in the patients with versus without OH, whereas albumin and 25-hydroxy vitamin D levels were significantly lower [9]. In addition, vitamin D deficiency has been shown in a meta-analysis in which OH is associated [10, 11].

All these results support that, besides age-related changes, many other factors can cause OH or increase complications related to OH [12, 13].

4. Are multiple organs affected?

A number of studies have reported associations between OH and increased risk of adverse clinical outcomes, including cardiovascular events and stroke, recurrent falls, syncope, and consequent injuries, cognitive impairment, impaired sleep quality, and depression. However, no attempt has been made to synthesize the literature on the health risks associated with OH or critically evaluate the strength of the available evidence. A better understanding of the full spectrum of health risks associated with OH is important for geriatric practice. For this purpose, an umbrella review published in 2019 containing 12 meta-analyses sheds light on the subject. In this review, there was suggestive evidence that OH was associated with significantly higher risk of coronary heart disease (HR = 1.32), stroke (HR = 1.22), congestive heart failure (HR = 1.30), all-cause mortality (RR = 1.50), falls (OR = 1.84), and dementia (HR = 1.22). OH can, therefore, be considered as a new geriatric syndrome [14].

5. Can the clinic picture be mild and are atypical presentations frequent?

OH can be symptomatic or asymptomatic. In one study, 1/3 of the patients with severe OH (>60 mmHg decrease in systolic blood pressure) were found to be asymptomatic. In the Cardiovascular Health study, the prevalence of OH was found to be 18% in ≥65-year-old participants, while only 2% were considered symptomatic (they described dizziness upon standing up) [4]. In another study, it was shown that the elderly who had OH at first, third, and fifth minutes were asymptomatic by 86.2%, 86.7%, and 84%, respectively [9].For this reason, it is appropriate to search for atypical signs and symptoms in cases suspected for the detection of asymptomatic cases, and to measure orthostatic blood pressure measurements of the patient at each visit. Although common signs and symptoms related to OH may be typical such as dizzinessand loss of balance, they can also be atypical such as fatigue, atypical nausea, paracervical pain, low back pain, angina pectoris, transient ischemic attack, visual impairment, speech impairment, syncope, falling, and cognitive impairment [15].All these signs and symptoms depend on the hypoperfusion of the relevant organ, as a result of temporary low blood pressure. The predictive value of these symptoms due to OH in the elderly is weak.

To sum up, OH may be a geriatric syndrome, as its frequency increases with age, multiple pathological and etiological factors play a role in the development of OH, it can be easily complicated, it affects multiple organ systems, and its clinic is often faint and can be presented with atypical symptoms.

References

1. Ates Bulut E, Soysal P, Isik AT. Frequency and coincidence of geriatric syndromes according to age groups: single-center experience in Turkey between 2013 and 2017. Clin Interv Aging. 2018;13:1899–905. https://doi.org/10.2147/CIA.S180281.
2. Mosnaim AD, Abiola R, Wolf ME, Perlmuter LC. Etiology and risk factors for developing orthostatic hypotension. Am J Ther. 2010;17(1):86–91. https://doi.org/10.1097/MJT.0b013e3181a2b1bb.
3. Low PA. Prevalence of orthostatic hypotension. Clin Auton Res. 2008;18(Suppl 1):8–13. https://doi.org/10.1007/s10286-007-1001-3.
4. Rutan GH, Hermanson B, Bild DE, Kittner SJ, LaBaw F, Tell GS. Orthostatic hypotension in older adults. The cardiovascular health study. CHS collaborative research group. Hypertension. 1992;19(6 Pt 1):508–19. https://doi.org/10.1161/01.hyp.19.6.508.
5. Joseph A, Wanono R, Flamant M, Vidal-Petiot E. Orthostatic hypotension: a review. Nephrol Ther. 2017;13(Suppl 1):S55–67. https://doi.org/10.1016/j.nephro.2017.01.003.
6. Gupta V, Lipsitz LA. Orthostatic hypotension in the elderly: diagnosis and treatment. Am J Med. 2007;120(10):841–7. https://doi.org/10.1016/j.amjmed.2007.02.023.
7. Poon IO, Braun U. High prevalence of orthostatic hypotension and its correlation with potentially causative medications among elderly veterans. J Clin Pharm Ther. 2005;30(2):173–8. https://doi.org/10.1111/j.1365-2710.2005.00629.x.
8. Pepersack T, Gilles C, Petrovic M, et al. Prevalence of orthostatic hypotension and relationship with drug use amongst older patients. Acta Clin Belg. 2013;68(2):107–12. https://doi.org/10.2143/ACB.3215.
9. Soysal P, Aydin AE, Koc Okudur S, Isik AT. When should orthostatic blood pressure changes be evaluated in elderly: 1st, 3rd or 5th minute? Arch Gerontol Geriatr. 2016;65:199–203. https://doi.org/10.1016/j.archger.2016.03.022.
10. Soysal P, Yay A, Isik AT. Does vitamin D deficiency increase orthostatic hypotension risk in the elderly patients? Arch Gerontol Geriatr. 2014;59(1):74–7. https://doi.org/10.1016/j.archger.2014.03.008.
11. Ometto F, Stubbs B, Annweiler C, et al. Hypovitaminosis D and orthostatic hypotension: a systematic review and meta-analysis. J Hypertens. 2016;34(6):1036–43. https://doi.org/10.1097/HJH.0000000000000907.
12. Kocyigit SE, Soysal P, Ates Bulut E, Isik AT. Malnutrition and malnutrition risk can be associated with systolic orthostatic hypotension in older adults. J Nutr Heal Aging. 2018;22(8):928–33. https://doi.org/10.1007/s12603-018-1032-6.

13. Kocyigit SE, Soysal P, Bulut EA, Aydin AE, Dokuzlar O, Isik AT. What is the relationship between frailty and orthostatic hypotension in older adults? J Geriatr Cardiol. 2019;16(3):272–9. https://doi.org/10.11909/j.issn.1671-5411.2019.03.005.
14. Soysal P, Veronese N, Smith L, et al. Orthostatic hypotension and health outcomes: an umbrella review of observational studies. Eur Geriatr Med. 2019; https://doi.org/10.1007/s41999-019-00239-4.
15. Fedorowski A, Melander O. Syndromes of orthostatic intolerance: a hidden danger. J Intern Med. 2013;273(4):322–35. https://doi.org/10.1111/joim.12021.

Epidemiology and Risk Factors Associated with Orthostatic Hypotension in Older Adults

3

Igor Grabovac, Galateja Jordakieva, and Lin Yang

Orthostatic hypotension, also called postural hypotension, is defined as a fall in blood pressure of at least 20 mmHg systolic or 10 mmHg diastolic caused by a change in posture, such as standing or tilt-testing [1]. It is often characterized as a dynamic state rather than a specific pathological entity and is a key manifestation of dysfunction of the autonomic system. Epidemiologic studies worldwide assessing the prevalence of orthostatic hypotension cite a wide range of proportions anywhere between 6% and 35% [2]. These estimates are a reflection of the variety of age and composition of the participants included in these studies as it has been reported that the prevalence of orthostatic hypotension rises with age and is associated with comorbidities and use of certain types of medication. Furthermore, orthostatic hypotension is associated with a variety of health outcomes such as syncope and falls, leading to functional impairments. Therefore, identifying the prevalence and associated risk factors is important in order to reduce the burden on patients and the health care systems.

I. Grabovac (✉)
Department of Social and Preventive Medicine, Centre for Public Health, Medical University of Vienna, Vienna, Austria
e-mail: igor.grabovac@meduniwien.ac.at

G. Jordakieva
Department of Physical Medicine, Rehabilitation and Occupational Medicine, Medical University of Vienna, Vienna, Austria
e-mail: galateja.jordakieva@meduniwien.ac.at

L. Yang
Department of Cancer Epidemiology and Prevention Research, Cancer Care Alberta, Alberta Health Services, Calgary, Canada

Departments of Oncology and Community Health Sciences, University of Calgary, Calgary, Canada

© Springer Nature Switzerland AG 2021
A. T. Isik, P. Soysal (eds.), *Orthostatic Hypotension in Older Adults*,
https://doi.org/10.1007/978-3-030-62493-4_3

3.1   Epidemiology

There are a number of studies giving reliable estimates of the prevalence of orthostatic hypotension with a high fluctuation in the reported results ranging from 5% to
35%. These differences vary based on the age of the population in question and the
presence of comorbidities (orthostatic hypotension is traditionally associated with
neurodegenerative diseases, frailty syndrome, chronic heart failure, diabetes mellitus, and arterial hypertension). Studies seem to unequivocally show that the prevalence of orthostatic hypotension rises with age. An US-based study on 557 healthy
subjects aged 10–83 years evenly distributed among age groups and gender reported
the overall prevalence of orthostatic hypotension at 5% also noting the rising prevalence with rising age [3]. A study on normotensive middle-aged adults in Sweden
reported a prevalence of 5.5%, with the same study reporting 13.4% prevalence in
those with hypertension [4].

A study of Indonesian adults aged over 40 years reported a prevalence of 12.6%
(mean age of those with orthostatic hypotension was 54 years) [5]. Similar results
were reported from a Chinese sample of community dwelling older adults (65 years
and over) with an orthostatic hypotension prevalence of 11% [6]. A study by Raiha
et al. on Finnish older adults aged 65 and older showed a prevalence of 28%; with a
later study on a random sample of Finnish older adults over 75 years reported the
prevalence of orthostatic hypotension at 34% [7, 8]. A study by Strogatz et al.
reported that in a sample of adults over 60 years, 12% of participants had a drop of
10 mmHg or more in systolic blood pressure when going from sitting to standing
position, furthermore reporting that the prevalence of orthostatic hypotension was
twice as more common among Caucasian comparing to African American participants (14.5% vs. 7.5%). The difference between the groups persisted even after
adjusting for weight status, medication, and other risk factors [9]. Overall, a recent
systematic review and meta-analysis on the prevalence of orthostatic hypotension
reported the pooled prevalence of orthostatic hypotension in community-dwelling
older people is 22.2% and somewhat more in those in long-term care settings at
23.9% [10]. However the strength of these evidence is influenced by various ways
of how orthostatic hypotension was assessed, despite clear guidelines. The authors
noted that the high variability between included studies did not allow for post-hoc
sensitivity analyses by various assessment methods.

3.2   Pathophysiology

Orthostatic hypotension results from at least one dysfunction in the chain of adaptive mechanisms essential to blood pressure regulation. Under physiological conditions, specialized mechanoreceptor (baroreceptor) cells, located in the aortic arch
and the carotid sinus, sense changes in blood pressure by the stretch of the blood
vessels walls. They transmit their sensory signals to the central nervous system,
specifically to the medulla oblongata, i.e., the brain stem, which in turn adapts cardiac output and systemic vascular resistance by regulation of smooth muscle

activity. Changing the body's posture from a lying to an upright position induces a gravity-related shift of approximately 500 ml of blood into the lower extremities, an effect known as venous pooling. The resulting acute decline of venous blood reflux and thus ventricular filling temporary reduces cardiac output by 20% and results in an immediate drop of systemic blood pressure. The direct consequence is an induced decrease in sympathetic, or vagal, nerve activity triggered by the brain stem. The results are chronotropic and inotropic effects on the heart muscle and an increase on peripheral vascular resistance, mediated by α1-adrenergic vasoconstriction of peripheral venous and splanchnic vessels and activation of the blood pressure regulating renoarterial renin and angiotensin II system. An adequate circulatory reaction leads to immediate blood pressure regulation and stabilization of cardiac output and, in consequence, cerebral blood supply. In short, several cardiovascular and neurological mechanisms are necessary to maintain hemodynamic properties and ensure a sufficient blood circulation. Any failure of these adaptive mechanisms or any factor contributing to their dysfunction poses a risk for the development, exacerbation, and/or maintaining of orthostatic hypotension. While a physiological age-dependent degeneration can be observed regarding these mechanisms, several of the most common risk factors are reversible. Elderly patients typically present with a combination of these risk factors or even occurrence of rare conditions, which sometimes raises the need for an interdisciplinary diagnostical approach. As a first step, common risk factors (detailed in Sect. 3.3), such as dehydration and drug-related orthostatic hypotension, must be excluded. If none of these can be identified or if a complex combination of underlying causes are suspected, an in-depth neurological and internal medical evaluation should be considered as a next step [11].

3.3 Risk Factors

3.3.1 Age as a Risk Factor for Orthostatic Hypotension

Orthostatic hypotension is a common condition in individuals over the age of 65 years, with a reported prevalence of up to 30%. The aforementioned age-dependent degradation of neuronal and vascular structures involved in the postural adaptive reaction includes impairments of the vestibulo-sympathetic reflex, diastolic filling capacity, chronotropic and inotropic cardiac responses, and vasoconstrictive abilities. While even a diminished baroreceptor sensitivity is discussed by some authors, several studies found that basal sympathetic activity increases with age. Besides the known physiological changes, the accumulation of other risk factors, such as blood pressure compromising comorbidities, progressed atherosclerosis of the cardiovascular and cerebral vessels, acute and chronic illnesses (e.g., neuropathies, diabetes mellitus), and multi-medication, results in a general increase in the prevalence of orthostatic hypotension over time. Also, a reduction in physical and daily living activity is significantly associated with orthostatic hypotension in older adults. A cross-sectional study on sex-specific differences in the prevalence of orthostatic hypotension showed no significant variations among women and men between 55 and 74, but a relative increase in prevalence after the age of 75 years, particularly in affected older women (30% versus 11% in men). Here, only systolic BP ≥ 140 mmHg was identified as a sex-specific risk factor for female hypotension, while BMI showed an inverse association with the prevalence of postural hypotension in both sexes [12]. The results may be somewhat biased as men may die before orthostatic hypotension could be diagnosed.

3.3.2 General and Lifestyle-Related Risk Factors

These include dehydration, deconditioning due to prolonged bed rest, postprandial hypotension, or mediation use.

1. Dehydration in older adults may result from insufficient intake or restrictive drinking or eating disorders, or from loss of water due to fever, sweating, alcohol consumptions, diarrhea, vomiting, and hemorrhageas well as heat exposure. Inadequate fluid intake but also significant loss of electrolytes and body water can lead to dehydration, which can further result in hypovolemia, i.e.,intravascular volume deficiency. In elderly patients whose oral fluid intake is latently insufficient, even mild dehydration can result in symptomatic orthostatic hypotension. In terms of intravascular volume loss, common mechanisms are fever, vomiting, diarrhea, or excessive sweating. Latter has to be considered particularly in excessive physical exercise and heat exposure. In addition, alcohol consumption can also result in dehydration by inhibition of anti-diuretic hormone release from the pituitary gland and decreased reabsorption of primary urine by the kidneys. Rare reasons for hypovolemia are hemorrhage and eating disorders (i.e., bulimia and anorexia nervosa). In elderly patients it is not uncommon for several of those causes to result in dehydration, adding up to induce symptomatic hypovolemia [13].
2. Prolonged bed rest due to illness or injury may lead to deconditioning. Gravitational stress, i.e., the change of posture from lying down to getting up, is the common trigger of postural adaptive mechanisms and might unmask orthostatic hypotension derived by other risk factors. It should be noted that in this context, even a slight delay in blood pressure regulation could be experienced as light-headedness upon rising, in the sense of an initial (transient) orthostatic hypotension. Upon longer bed rest, however, intravascular volume is gradually redistributed, sympathetic nerve activity diminished and, over time, even the cardiovascular system adapts to the lack of gravitational stress, resulting in deconditioning and orthostatic hypotension upon getting up again [14, 15]. A study in heart failure patients, for example, showed a significant increase in orthostatic hypotension risk with each hour of lying down [16]. In cases of long-term bed rest over several weeks, additionally an impairment of the vestibulo-sympathetic reflex was found to contribute to postural orthostatic dysfunction [17]. If the bed rest is resulted from illness, several auxiliary risk factors, e.g., dehydration and medication, can concur and aggravate the orthostatic hypotension induced by deconditioning.

3. Postprandial hypotension (low blood pressure after eating meals) is commonly observed in elderly patients. In an acute geriatric ward, postprandial hypotension, particularly in the first 75 min after a meal, was shown to affect almost 50% of patients, and found to coincide with orthostatic hypotension in one-third of those who also had orthostatic hypotension [18].

4. Medication use is the most common risk factors for orthostatic hypotension. Particularly substances for hypertensive blood pressure regulation with vasoactive and pro-diuretic effects may cause orthostatic hypertension alone or in combination, even with over-the-counter products. An early study in 50 elderly patients identified diuretics (56%), benzodiazepines (26%), antidepressants (24%), and anti-Parkinson drugs (22%) as the most common iatrogenic causes of orthostatic hypotension. Out of all diuretic drugs, the anti-aldosterone spironolactone, which leads to impaired renal water and sodium reabsorption, has been most frequently associated with orthostatic hypotension. Another common drug frequently reported to cause orthostatic hypotension in older patients is the loop-diuretic furosemide and thiazide diuretics, which has proved especially problematic in elderly patients with concomitant heart failure. Calcium channel blockers, particularly non-dihydropyridine, additionally exhibit negative inotropic and dromotropic myocardial effects, resulting in a 2–5-fold increase in orthostatic hypotension risk in elderly patients. Alpha1-blockers, like doxazosin, directly inhibit vasoconstriction but also affect cardiac output and baroreceptor activity leading to postural hypotonia, particularly in settings of hypovolemia. Beta-blockers may impair the postural compensatory mechanisms in older individuals by reducing activity of the renal renin-angiotensin system. While both ACE inhibitors and angiotensin II receptor antagonists are associated with pertinent hemodynamic effects, their role in orthostatic hypotension is still controversial. Parkinson's disease can, on one hand, directly induce autonomic dysfunction and, on the other hand, indirectly promote postural hypotension through the side effects of anti-Parkinson medication, in particular dopaminergic agonists like levodopa. The combination with selegiline appears to further heighten the adverse effects of vasodilation and sympathetic activity reduction. As no dose-dependent effects have been identified in this context, however, it is suspected that these medications alone do not cause orthostatic dysregulation but support its manifestation in settings with other risk factors, particularly multi-medication. While less commonly associated with orthostatic hypotension, sedatives have been shown to reduce myocardial contractility, central vasomotor as well as peripheral vascular activity. The benzodiazepine temazepam has been associated with hypotensive reactions. However, data is inconsistent in terms on effects of sedatives in the elderly. Similarly, anesthetics, especially propofol, impact cardiac contractility, sinus node polarization, and arterial vasodilation with both dose- and concentration-dependent induction of orthostatic dysfunction. Tricyclic antidepressants are well known to induce hypotension by alpha receptor blockade. Further, even serotonin-uptake inhibitors have been shown to enhance vasodilatation through calcium channel inhibition and contribute to postural blood pressure dysregulation. Fluoxetine additionally exhibits effects

on the central nervous system in favor of orthostatic hypotension. While also associated with postural hypotension, data on antipsychotics and atypical neuroleptics is limited. Peripheral vasodilatation and reduction of vasomotor reflexes by opioid analgesics is also a less common iatrogenic risk factor, but has been shown to promote hypotension in elderly patients with hypovolemia. Phosphodiesterase-5 inhibitors, like sildenafil, may exacerbate neurodegenerative conditions in elderly patients with primary autonomic dysregulation and particularly exacerbate the effects of nitrates. Several other substances have been associated with orthostatic hypotension; the desired mechanisms of these drugs are often associated with vasodilatation or sympathetic nervous system disruption, whereas for other drug classes the mechanism of action still remains unclear [19].

3.3.3 Medical Conditions as Risk Factors

These conditions are often classified as either neurogenic or non-neurogenic (cardiac, endocrine, metabolic) forms and may influence occurrence of orthostatic hypotension (Table 3.1).

Table 3.1 Medical conditions as risk factors of orthostatic hypotension

System	Conditions
Cardiovascular	Cardiac disorders: • Disorders ofthe heart valves • Myocardial infarction • Congestive heart failure • Myocarditis • Pericarditis • Arrhythmic disorders Vascular conditions: • Atherosclerosis • Vasculitis
Neurologic	Primary autonomic failure: • Parkinson's disease with autonomic failure • Multiple system atrophy • Pure autonomic failure Secondary autonomic failure: • Peripheral neuropathies (acute and subacute, acute and paraneoplastic pandysautonomia, Guillain–Barré syndrome, diabetes mellitus, amyloidosis, hereditary illnesses, Sjörgen's syndrome, heavy metal and other toxicity, porphyria, and other peripheral neuropathies as a result of infections, connective tissue diseases,and metabolic nutritional issues)
Metabolic-endocrine	• Diabetes mellitus • Thyroid diseases • Adrenal insufficiency (Addison's disease and diabetes insipidus) • Hypoglycemia • Vitamins B_{12} and D deficiency • Pheochromocytoma

1. As the heart is central to hemodynamic regulation, a failure to provide sufficient volume output, e.g., due to mechanical restrictions, i.e., valve disorders and left-ventricular hypertrophy [20], or due to myocardial dysfunction, resulting from post-infarction areas and inflammation, is a significant risk factor for the failure of an adequate orthostatic response [21]. Co-existence of heart failure and orthostatic hypotension is particularly common among elderly patients, estimated to manifest in 8–12% community dwelling and 23–33% hospitalized older adults. Additionally, arrhythmia leading to significant changes in cardiac output, most prominently bradycardia, can also impair hemodynamic stability, particularly upon exposing to gravitational stress [22]. Age-related loss of vascular compliance, commonly referred to as "arterial stiffness," dampens the hemodynamic response in the postural phase. Firstly, the limited arterial elasticity results in an impairment of baroreceptor sensitivity and subsequent sympathetic activation. Secondly, arterial stiffness directly restricts the vasoconstricting potential of the affected vessels. In the elderly with a lack of physical exercise, vascular compliance has been described as particularly impaired [23]. Although a relatively rare occurrence, inflammation of the large arterial vessels, e.g., in case of Takayasu's arteritis, can also diminish baroreceptor function [24].

2. Neurodegenerative disorders impairing the regulatory capacity of the autonomic nervous system are common contributors to orthostatic dysregulation in elderly patients. In pure autonomic failure, a condition commonly manifesting with orthostatic hypotension, slowly progressive autonomic nervous degeneration, without other neurological involvement, has been observed. The suspected underlying cause is neuronal α-synuclein deposition, a pathological mechanism, which can gradually lead to severe neurodegenerative conditions, such as multisystem atrophy, dementia with Lewy bodies or Parkinson's disease. The latter leads to an age-related increase in orthostatic hypotension incidence, which has a clear association with Parkinson's disease severity and duration [25]. The prevalence of postural hypotension is estimated to be around 50% in Parkinson and in Dementia with Lewy bodies, respectively. In multisystem atrophy, a neurodegenerative disorder with autonomic dysfunction, and cerebellar ataxia, a prevalence of postural hypotension up to 75% is reported. All three conditions are further associated with the impairment of norepinephrine release in approximately two-thirds of affected patients, which limits peripheral vascular resistance, venous reflux, and autonomic regulation of the myocardium. In contrast to the aforementioned primary causes of autonomic nerve degeneration, a wide range of non-neurological diseases, e.g., amyloidosis, inflammatory and autoimmune diseases, vitamin deficiencies, uremia, and diabetes mellitus as well as toxic substances, such as certain chemotherapeutic agents and heavy metals, can lead to nonselective neuropathies. These conditions may also affect central sympathetic activity and are thus classified as secondary autonomic nervous system diseases in the context of orthostatic hypotension [26].

3. As already mentioned above, diabetes mellitus and the resulting diabetic polyneuropathy are metabolic conditions commonly associated with orthostatic hypotension, where higher HbA1c levels are found among affected patients. The

prevalence of orthostatic hypotension is estimated to be around 6% in diabetes mellitus type I and around 7% in type II diabetes mellitus, with the prevalence rising to 23% in patients with diabetic neuropathy [27]. A dysregulation of thyroid function manifesting with hypothyreotic metabolic state often results in a drop in blood pressure and may further predispose to a manifestation of orthostatic hypotension [28, 29]. Similarly, adrenal insufficiency, as seen in Addison's disease and in diabetes insipidus patients, leads to dysregulations of systemic electrolyte and body water management, as well as to autonomic dysfunction [30, 31]. Recently, vitamin D deficiency has been investigated as a potential risk factor in the development of orthostatic hypotension. The suspected underlying mechanism is a dysfunction of vascular and endothelial smooth muscle cells due to a lack of the active 25(OH) vitamin D. An evaluation and correction of serum vitamin levels, particularly vitamin D but also B_{12}, should be considered in elderly patients with restricted everyday physical and nutritional activities [32]. While one of the less common risk factors, pheochromocytoma has been found to manifest orthostatic hypotension in two-thirds of cases, due to dysregulated increases in plasma norepinephrine concentrations [33]. A similar dysregulation of catecholamine responses appears to be a relevant pathological mechanism during hypoglycemia [34]. Interestingly, orthostatic hypotension has been frequently identified in patients with renal failure, leading to independent associations with quality of life, adverse health effects, including falls and fractures, and mortality in hemodialysis patients. Besides disturbances in the renin-angiotensin blood pressure regulation, a concomitant severe anemia, which is commonly observed in chronic kidney disease patients due to limitations in renal erythropoietin production, might contribute to postural hypotension [35, 36].

In summary, a highly functioning loop of circulatory regulation mechanisms is required to maintain a stable blood pressure after changing posture from a horizontal into an upright position. Factors impairing adequate venous reflux, circulation of effective blood volume, baroreceptor activation, sympathetic and parasympathetic as well as cardiovascular adrenoreceptor (α- and β) activity and vasoconstriction all result in an increased likelihood of orthostatic hypotension [37]. While several conditions like anxiety, panic disorder, and shock might mimic orthostatic dysregulation, they are rather differential diagnoses than risk factors. While a multitude of risk factors are associated with orthostatic hypotension, orthostatic hypotension itself is a risk factor for adverse health outcomes. Based on the associated decline of cerebral and myocardial blood supply, orthostatic hypotension can act as an independent risk factor for cardiovascular morbidity and mortality in coronary artery disease and stroke [38]. These findings further stress the importance of adequate recognition and eliminating risk factors of postural hypotension in elderly patients, supplemented with timely diagnosis and treatment.

3.3.4   Orthostatic Hypotension as Predictor for Other Health Outcomes

Growing evidence suggests that orthostatic hypotension and other disorders of postural hemodynamic control predict all-cause mortality and the incidence of cardiovascular disease with the same, if not better, accuracy than outpatient-based measurements showing night time reverse dipping [39–43]. Additionally, some studies have also noted that in longitudinal observations, orthostatic hypotension is a risk factor of cause-specific mortality for patients diagnosed with stroke and cardiovascular disease; however the evidence supporting this is not consistent across reported studies [41, 44, 45]. Nevertheless, a 2015 meta-analysis of 13 studies encompassing more than 120,000 patients with a median follow up time of 6 years reported that orthostatic hypotension was associated with higher risk of all-cause mortality, as well as incident coronary heart disease, heart failure, and stroke. Pooled estimates, interestingly, showed higher risk ratios for patients under 65 years of age compared to older ones [46]. Authors concluded that there was a need for more studies, given the limitations in heterogeneousmeasurements and study populations. Similar to this meta-analysis, other population-based studies also reported that the relative risk of orthostatic hypotension predicted stroke mortality decreasedas age increased [47]. The prospective results of the Malmö Preventive Project also reported that those who were under 42 years and had orthostatic hypotension were at a two-fold higher risk of death [48].

Overall the potential mechanism that explains the link between orthostatic hypotension and negative outcomes has been proposed; however it requires several considerations; namely higher variability of blood pressure during the day as well as nocturnal hypertension which are usually present in patients with orthostatic hypotension may provoke spells of increased cardiac afterload leading to ventricular hypertrophy and decreased renal function, ultimately leading to congestive heart failure and ischemia. Moreover, Fedorowski et al. reported that, independent of all usual risk factors, the incidence of atrial fibrillation was higher among people who had arterial hypertension and orthostatic hypotension, which further strengthens the evidence supporting a link between orthostatic hypotension and cardiovascular morbidity [49]. Furthermore, orthostatic hypotension seems to also activate the neuroendocrine compensatory mechanisms leading to the hyper-activationendothelin system. As such vasoconstrictors may promote thrombotic effects leading to further cerebro-cardiovascular morbidity and mortality, it is important to note that these hypotheses have not yet been confirmed and that there is still no firm consensus on the causal links. In other words, it is still unknown if orthostatic hypotension is an independent general marker of death or an intermediate variable operating within a (higher-order) pathomechanistic response. Most authors concur that more epidemiologic studies should be encouraged.

References

1. American Autonomic Society and American Academy of Neurology. Consensus statement on the definition of orthostatic hypotension, pure autonomic failure, and multiple system atrophy. The consensus Committee of the American Autonomic Society and the American Academy of Neurology. Neurology. 1996;46(5):1470.
2. Ricci F, De Caterina R, Fedorowski A. Orthostatic hypotension: Epidemiology, Prognosis, and Treatment. J Am Coll Cardiol. 2015;66(7):848–60.
3. Low PA, et al. Effect of age and gender on sudomotor and cardiovagal function and blood pressure response to tilt in normal subjects. Muscle Nerve. 1997;20(12):1561–8.
4. Fedorowski A, Burri P, Melander O. Orthostatic hypotension in genetically related hypertensive and normotensive individuals. J Hypertens. 2009;27(5):976–82.
5. Siti S, Bambang S, Wiguno P. The prevalence of orthostatic hypotension and its risk factors among 40 years and above adult population in Indonesia. Med J Indonesia. 2004;13(3):20–5.
6. Zhu QO, et al. Orthostatic hypotension: prevalence and associated risk factors among the ambulatory elderly in an Asian population. Singap Med J. 2016;57(8):444–51.
7. Hiitola P, et al. Postural changes in blood pressure and the prevalence of orthostatic hypotension among home-dwelling elderly aged 75 years or older. J Hum Hypertens. 2009;23(1):33–9.
8. Räihä I, et al. Prevalence, predisposing factors, and prognostic importance of postural hypotension. Arch Intern Med. 1995;155(9):930–5.
9. Strogatz DS, et al. Correlates of postural hypotension in a community sample of elderly blacks and whites. J Am Geriatr Soc. 1991;39(6):562–6.
10. Saedon NI, Pin Tan M, Frith J. The prevalence of orthostatic hypotension: a systematic review and meta-analysis. J Gerontol A Biol Sci Med Sci. 2020;75(1):117–22.
11. Braune S, Lücking CH. Orthostatische hypotonie: pathophysiologie, differentialdiagnose und therapie. Dtsch Arztebl Int. 1997;94(50):3413.
12. Mendez AS, et al. Risk factors for orthostatic hypotension: differences between elderly men and women. Am J Hypertens. 2018;31(7):797–803.
13. Lavizzo-Mourey RJ. Dehydration in the elderly: a short review. J Natl Med Assoc. 1987;79(10):1033–8.
14. Kamiya A, et al. Pathophysiology of orthostatic hypotension after bed rest: paradoxical sympathetic withdrawal. Am J Phys Heart Circ Phys. 2003;285(3):H1158–67.
15. Parsaik A, et al. Deconditioning in patients with orthostatic intolerance. Neurology. 2012;79(14):1435–9.
16. Gorelik O, et al. Seating-induced postural hypotension is common in older patients with decompensated heart failure and may be prevented by lower limb compression bandaging. Gerontology. 2009;55(2):138–44.
17. Dyckman DJ, Sauder CL, Ray CA. Effects of short-term and prolonged bed rest on the vestibulosympathetic reflex. Am J Physiol Heart Circ Physiol. 2012;302(1):H368–74.
18. Schoevaerdts D, et al. Prevalence and risk factors of postprandial hypotension among elderly people admitted in a geriatric evaluation and management unit : an observational study. J Nutr Health Aging. 2019;23(10):1026–33.
19. Milazzo V, et al. Drugs and orthostatic hypotension: evidence from literature. Journal of Hypertension. 2012;1(2):1–8.
20. Fan X-H, et al. Disorders of orthostatic blood pressure response are associated with cardiovascular disease and target organ damage in hypertensive patients. Am J Hypertens. 2010;23(8):829–37.
21. Gorelik O, Feldman L, Cohen N. Heart failure and orthostatic hypotension. Heart Fail Rev. 2016;21(5):529–38.
22. Gupta R, et al. Symptomatic bradycardia and postural hypotension. Postgrad Med J. 2004;80(949):679–81.
23. Boddaert J, et al. Arterial stiffness is associated with orthostatic hypotension in elderly subjects with history of falls. J Am Geriatr Soc. 2004;52(4):568–72.

24. Habermann CR, Münzel T. Takayasu's arteritis. Lancet. 2001;358(9287):1050.
25. Ha AD, et al. The prevalence of symptomatic orthostatic hypotension in patients with Parkinson's disease and atypical parkinsonism. Parkinsonism Relat Disord. 2011;17(8):625–8.
26. Coon EA, Singer W, Low PA. Pure Autonomic Failure. Mayo Clin Proc. 2019;94(10):2087–98.
27. Winkler A, Bosman D. Symptomatic postural hypotension in diabetes: aetiology and management. Pract Diabet Int. 2003;20(6):219–25.
28. Blum I, Barkan A, Yeshurun D. Thyrotoxicosis presenting as orthostatic hypotension. Postgrad Med J. 1980;56(656):425.
29. Lambert M, et al. Orthostatic hypotension associated with hypothyroidism. Acta Clin Belg. 1984;39(1):48–50.
30. Barbot M, et al. Cardiovascular autonomic dysfunction in patients with idiopathic diabetes insipidus. Pituitary. 2018;21(1):50–5.
31. Papierska L, Rabijewski M. Delay in diagnosis of adrenal insufficiency is a frequent cause of adrenal crisis. Int J Endocrinol. 2013;2013:482370.
32. Schroeder C, Jordan J, Kaufmann H. Management of neurogenic orthostatic hypotension in patients with autonomic failure. Drugs. 2013;73(12):1267–79.
33. Streeten DHP, Anderson GH. Mechanisms of orthostatic hypotension and tachycardia in patients with Pheochromocytoma*. Am J Hypertens. 1996;9(8):760–9.
34. Polinsky RJ, et al. The adrenal medullary response to hypoglycemia in patients with orthostatic hypotension. J Clin Endocrinol Metabol. 1980;51(6):1401–6.
35. Liu W, et al. Impaired orthostatic blood pressure stabilization and reduced hemoglobin in chronic kidney disease. J Clin Hypertension. 2019;21(9):1317–24.
36. Soysal P, Yay A, Isik AT. Does vitamin D deficiency increase orthostatic hypotension risk in the elderly patients? Arch Gerontol Geriatr. 2014;59(1):74–7.
37. Mosnaim AD, et al. Etiology and risk factors for developing orthostatic hypotension. Am J Ther. 2010;17(1):86–91.
38. Schimpf R, Veltmann C, Borggrefe M. Orthostatic hypotension : diagnosis and therapy. Herzschrittmacherther Elektrophysiol. 2011;22(2):99–106.
39. Eigenbrodt ML, et al. Orthostatic hypotension as a risk factor for stroke: the atherosclerosis risk in communities (ARIC) study, 1987-1996. Stroke. 2000;31(10):2307–13.
40. Fagard RH, De Cort P. Orthostatic hypotension is a more robust predictor of cardiovascular events than nighttime reverse dipping in elderly. Hypertension. 2010;56(1):56–61.
41. Masaki KH, et al. Orthostatic hypotension predicts mortality in elderly men: the Honolulu heart program. Circulation. 1998;98(21):2290–5.
42. Sasaki O, et al. Orthostatic hypotension at the introductory phase of haemodialysis predicts all-cause mortality. Nephrol Dial Trans. 2004;20(2):377–81.
43. Verwoert GC, et al. Orthostatic hypotension and risk of cardiovascular disease in elderly people: the Rotterdam study. J Am Geriatr Soc. 2008;56(10):1816–20.
44. Hossain M, Ooi WL, Lipsitz LA. Intra-individual postural blood pressure variability and stroke in elderly nursing home residents. J Clin Epidemiol. 2001;54(5):488–94.
45. Weiss A, et al. Influence of orthostatic hypotension on mortality among patients discharged from an acute geriatric ward. J Gen Intern Med. 2006;21(6):602–6.
46. Ricci F, et al. Cardiovascular morbidity and mortality related to orthostatic hypotension: a meta-analysis of prospective observational studies. Eur Heart J. 2015;36(25):1609–17.
47. Rose KM, et al. Orthostatic hypotension predicts mortality in middle-aged adults: the atherosclerosis risk in communities (ARIC) study. Circulation. 2006;114(7):630–6.
48. Fedorowski A, et al. Orthostatic hypotension predicts all-cause mortality and coronary events in middle-aged individuals (the Malmo preventive project). Eur Heart J. 2010;31(1):85–91.
49. Fedorowski A, et al. Orthostatic hypotension and long-term incidence of atrial fibrillation: the malmö preventive project. J Intern Med. 2010;268(4):383–9.

Orthostatic Hypotension: Clinical Features

4

Esra Ates Bulut ⓘ and Bilgin Comert ⓘ

4.1   Orthostatic Hypotension: Clinical Features

Orthostatic hypotension (OH), defined as a sustained reduction in systolic blood pressure (SBP) of at least 20 mmHg or diastolic blood pressure (DBP) of 10 mmHg within 3 min of standing or head-up tilt (HUT), is frequent observation in older adults [1–3]. Prevalence of postural hypotension which varies between the studies because of the difference in the methodology used, was reported to range from 9% to 30% in older-aged community-dwelling adults and increases to more than 50% in hospitalized geriatric patients [4]. Stabilization of postural change in blood pressure (BP) requires complex physiological functions, coordinated by the interaction between cardiovascular, renal, neuromuscular, and endocrine systems. OH is a complex syndrome, and often multifactorial as well. OH may be classified into neurogenic or non-neurogenic OH according to pathophysiologic mechanisms. Neurogenic OH is mainly reported in patients with primary neurodegenerative diseases called α-synucleinopathies [5], and diabetes mellitus, multiple sclerosis, demyelinating polyneuropathies, brainstem and spinal cord lesions, as that diseases affect the autonomic nervous system. On the other hand, non-neurogenic OH may be developed because of volume depletion, medications, heart failure, and venous pooling [6]. Accordingly, age-related diminished physiological reserve, loss of baroreceptor sensitivity, increased arterial stiffness, autonomic dysfunction, systemic diseases, sarcopenia and drugs blunt the compensatory response to orthostatic challenge. Older patients, especially using vasoactive hypotensive drugs, and diagnosed with hypertension, cardiovascular disease are susceptible to orthostatic stress.

E. Ates Bulut (✉)
Department of Geriatric Medicine, Adana State Training and Research Hospital, Adana, Turkey

B. Comert
Department of Internal Medicine, Division of Medical Intensive Care, Dokuz Eylul University, Faculty of Medicine, Izmir, Turkey

© Springer Nature Switzerland AG 2021
A. T. Isik, P. Soysal (eds.), *Orthostatic Hypotension in Older Adults*,
https://doi.org/10.1007/978-3-030-62493-4_4

Patients with hypertension are more vulnerable to cerebral ischemia even for a short-term period because of alteration in the cerebral autoregulation due to the chronic blood pressure elevation. Moreover, lower blood pressure targets and tight blood pressure control may also contribute to adverse health outcomes such as falls in conjunction with OH [7]. Other risk factors for OH include age, smoking, low body mass index, malnutrition, renal dysfunction, autoimmune diseases, and cancer [8, 9]. Higher prevalence, and larger drop in systolic blood pressure have been found to be associated with increasing age and physical frailty [10, 11]. Furthermore, hypertension, heart failure, Parkinson's disease, diabetes mellitus, chronic kidney disease, significant accompanying chronic conditions with OH, are the major risk factors for cardiovascular disease at the same time.

In this chapter, we review the clinical manifestations of OH according to underlying pathophysiologic mechanisms, and current understanding of the relation between OH and clinical outcomes.

4.1.1   Orthostatic Intolerance and Orthostatic Hypotension

The term "orthostatic intolerance (OI)" is used to describe symptoms and signs which are manifested with standing up that are relieved by recumbency. As a definition, symptoms should initiate when standing [12]. OI is not always due to autonomic or other compensatory mechanism dysfunction and can be due to insufficiency of compensatory responses to environmental stressors. For example, transient OI is commonly encountered during dehydration or infectious disease.

Patients frequently present with dizziness, discomfort, nausea, palpitations, and sometimes loss of consciousness. Some patients suffer from severe orthostatic intolerance symptoms without drop in blood pressure. OI is heterogeneous and multifactorial disorder, mainly classified as OH, postural orthostatic tachycardia syndrome (POTS), and orthostatic vasovagal syncope. POTS is caused by an inappropriate heart rate increase with upright posture and eventually causes light-headedness, palpitations, and fatigue without blood pressure decrease. Vasovagal reflex syncope is triggered by prolonged standing, pain or emotion leading to change in autonomic nervous system activity, cardiac depression and vasodilatation. Syncope is preceded by prodromal symptoms such as nausea, pallor, sweating [13].

Classical OH is defined as reduction of systolic blood pressure of at least 20 mmHg or diastolic blood pressure of 10 mmHg within 3 min of standing or head-up tilt to at least 60° on a tilt table [1]. Clinical variants of OH was determined as initial, classical, and delayed OH according to the consensus [1]. The blamed pathophysiologic mechanisms, and diagnostic criteria of each OH variant are summarized in the Table 4.1 [14]. The clinical manifestations of OH occur due to circulatory abnormality of the organs. The symptoms of OH may vary greatly upon severity of the hypoperfusion, patients may experience several symptoms including, light-headedness, dizziness, fainting, weakness, fatigue, cognitive difficulties, vision changes, head/neck pain, calf claudication, syncope even angina, which results in a reduced quality of life [15]. Symptoms including palpitation, tremor are seen due to sympathetic activity in patients whose autonomic functions remain intact. Several

Table 4.1 Characteristics of Orthostatic Hypotension Variants

OH	Time of BP measurement after standing	Drop in BP	Potential mechanisms
Initial	0–15 s	• ≥40 mmHg SBP and/or ≥20 mmHg DBP	• Transient mismatch between cardiac output and peripheral vascular resistance
Classic	15–180 s	• ≥20 mmHg SBP and/or ≥10 mmHg DBP or • ≥30 mmHg SBP in supine HT or a decrease in SBP to <90 mmHg	• Excessive fall of cardiac output • Defective inadequate vasoconstrictor mechanisms(autonomic instability)
Delayed	>3 min	• ≥20 mmHg SBP and/or ≥10 mmHg DBP or • ≥30 mmHg SBP in supine HT or • a decrease in SBP to <90 mmHg	• Mild or early form of sympathetic adrenergic failure • Defect in venous return

BP Blood Pressure, *HT* Hypertension, *OH* Orthostatic Hypotension, *SBP* Systolic Blood Pressure, *DBP* Diastolic Blood Pressure
Adapted from Freeman, et al. Consensus statement on the definition of orthostatic hypotension, neurally mediated syncope and the postural tachycardia syndrome [1]; Brignole, et al. 2018 ESC Guidelines for the diagnosis and management of syncope [2]; Fedorowski, et al. Syndromes of orthostatic intolerance: a hidden danger [14]

precipitating factors such as sudden positional change, prolonged recumbency, heat, meal, and physical strain have been described [10]. Specifically, symptoms are subsided in a seated or supine position.

4.1.2 Associated Clinical Features of Orthostatic Hypotension

Recent population studies support that vast majority of OH patients detected by screening or routine evaluation are asymptomatic [16]. Additionally, the underlying causes cannot be identified in almost one-third of the patients with persistent OH after an extensive evaluation [17]. Although many subjects are asymptomatic and OH is frequently overlooked by physicians, it places huge burden on healthcare system and is an important risk factor for hospitalization in older adults. Nationwide Inpatient Sample in the United States estimated hospitalization rate of 233 per 100,000 patients over 75 years of age, with a median length of stay of three days and an overall in-hospital mortality rate of 0.9% due to OH [18].

Patients, particularly with neurogenic OH, have also some other accompanying conditions which make difficult the management of the patients. Patients have commonly suffer from other dysautonomic symptoms including digestive disorders (diarrhea or constipation), urinary symptoms (urgency or atonic bladder), mydriasis, hypo- or hyperhidrosis, and erectile dysfunction [15]. Additionally, up to 50% of patients with OH, especially who has autonomic dysfunction, have supine

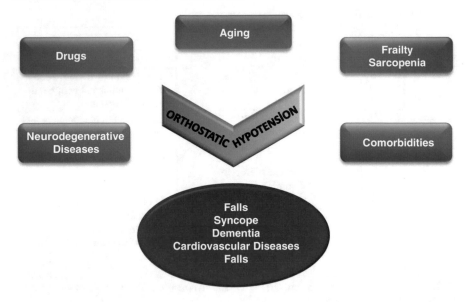

Fig. 4.1 Orthostatic hypotension in older adults

hypertension (systolic blood pressure >150 mmHg or diastolic blood pressure >90 mmHg while in the supine position) [19]. Supine hypertension requires some additional considerations. Supine hypertension restricts treatment options for OH and has been associated with a number of complications including impaired renal function and left ventricular hypertrophy [20]. Postprandial hypotension, commonly encountered in patients with primary or secondary autonomic failure, is a frequent cause of falls, syncope, and stroke [21]. Moreover, excessive pooled venous peripheral blood is redistributed to the central areas during the night in patients with OH. Nocturnal polyuria cause volume depletion, and redistribution of intravascular volume causes diurnal variability. Orthostatic blood pressure responses may not be reproducible in patients with documented OH symptoms, repeated blood pressure measurements may be needed to prove the diagnosis. Therefore, appropriate assessment of OH is advised to be done in the morning because of the high sensitivity [22].

OH not only has close relationship with debilitating diseases such as multiple system atrophy, amyloidosis, cancer, diabetes, but also carries poor prognosis in itself. Furthermore, emerging evidences have indicated that failure of blood pressure stabilization has been found to be associated with falls, syncope, depression, and global cognitive impairment [23–27], and is also critical to be functionally dependent. OH has been reported as a risk factor for cardiovascular and all-cause mortality, due to underlying causes and associated diseases [28].Risk factors and outcomes of OH are schematized in the Figure 4.1.

4.1.2.1 Falls and Syncope
Elderly people are susceptible to acute changes in cerebral blood flow, predisposing them to falls and syncope. Falls, most of which can be preventable, are the leading

cause of injury in older people [29]. OH is shown as an independent risk factor for future falls, unexplained falls, and injurious falls [30]. The effect of OH on brain and muscle microcirculation may contribute to falls [27]. Moreover, gait and balance difficulties, cognitive impairment, autonomic instability in patients with neurogenic OH create additional risk for falls. The association between OH and falls was strongest in the subgroup of studies using continuous blood pressure measurements, suggesting that testing OH with this method has the largest clinical relevance [26]. Consequently, the American Geriatrics Society Clinical Practice Guideline for Prevention of Falls in Older Persons suggests assessment and treatment of postural hypotension as a part of multifactorial intervention approach [31].

OH is a well-known risk factor for syncope, accounting as a cause in 24% of all diagnosed cases. Furthermore, patients with OH are older; have more comorbid conditions including hypertension, organic heart disease, and abnormal electrocardiogram; are taking more hypotensive medications; and require more frequent hospitalization [32]. Presence of neurodegenerative diseases, polypharmacy, malnutrition, peripheral neuropathies (e.g., diabetes mellitus) make significant contribution to development of orthostatic syncope. Orthostatic syncope was reported nearly 50% in patient samples diagnosed with dementia [5, 33]. Additionally, older persons with hypertension, cardiovascular disease or receiving vasoactive drugs whose circulatory compensatory adjustments to orthostatic stress are disturbed, are vulnerable to develop postural hypotension. Notably, dementia and hypertension coincidence is remarkable, and attention should be paid to hypertension treatment in demented patients. *Higher diastolic blood pressure drops in the orthostatic challenge and OH were reported to be associated with cognitive decline* [34]. *On the other hand, low blood pressure leading to c*erebral hypoperfusion could participate in the pathogenesis of cognitive decline [35]. Therefore, patients with advanced age and cognitive impairment should be assessed and managed on an individual basis.

4.1.2.2 Cognition

Cardiovascular disease and its risk factors were shown to be associated with cognitive decline and dementia. However, the results of conducted studies searching the potential causal relationship between OH and cognition remain inconclusive. Some hypotheses have been suggested to clarify the relation. One of that supports a common pathophysiologic mechanism affecting both cognition and cardiovascular autonomic control. Alternatively, OH may play role in cognitive decline with chronic cerebral hypoperfusion. Considering several disorders coexistence with OH, *identifying the cause* of cognitive impairment is difficult [36]. The Atherosclerosis Risk in Communities (ARIC) follow-up study for 6 years, showed no relation between OH and cognitive decline after multivariate adjustment [37]. However, OH was found to be independently associated with an increased risk of dementia and ischemic stroke during ≈25 years of follow-up of the ARIC study group [25]. The Irish Longitudinal Study on Ageing (TILDA), in which community-living non-stroke, non-demented, and non-Parkinsonian individuals were followed over 2 years, assessed cognitive functions using Mini-Mental State Exam (MMSE), verbal fluency, and word recall tasks. After adjustment of potential confounders, impairedrecovery of blood pressure at 40 s post standing was not found to be associated with change in performance on the aforementioned cognitive measures [38].

Furthermore, OH patterns may also differ according to the types and severity of dementia [5]. Regarding to OH, higher prevalence, and more significant and prolonged drop of systolic blood pressure were reported in the group of Dementia with Lewy bodies compared to Alzheimer's Disease [39]. Additionally, delayed OH may constitute a greater risk of cognitive decline or incident dementia than patients with early OH, as they are more likely to experience longer periods of cerebral hypoperfusion, and consequently ischemia [40]. In contrast to initial OH, delayed recovery from orthostatic blood pressure changes is reported as an increased risk for falls, cognitive impairment, and frailty [41]. Consequently, discrepancy between studies may be explained by the different methodology used and OH duration of patients, and insufficient sensitivity or specificity of screening tests to detect change in cognitive functions. Further studies are needed to elucidate the exact pathophysiologic mechanisms and effect of OH on cognitive functions.

4.1.2.3 Cardiovascular Disease and Mortality

The presence of OH independently predicts coronary events, stroke, heart failure, and CV mortality [42]. Although antihypertensive treatment is usually blamed as a risk factor for OH, researches show contradictive results. The HYTE (Hypertension Heredity in Malmö Evaluation) study cohort [43], the SPRINT [Systolic Blood Pressure Intervention Trial] [44] in individuals without stroke or diabetes, the ALLHAT (Antihypertensive and Lipid-Lowering Treatment to Prevent Heart Attack Trial) [45] a randomized clinical trial, and the AASK (African American Study of Kidney Disease) trial [46] in African Americans with chronic kidney disease (CKD) showed that antihypertensive medications may reduce or not affect the impaired orthostatic response. Although antihypertensive treatment seems to decrease OH, it may also increase the vasovagal reflex tendency and fall risk in vulnerable individuals. Therefore, it is important to consider identification of optimal personal blood pressure target in older adults in order to prevent unwanted health outcomes such as syncope, falls, and cardiovascular events.

Moreover, presence of cardiovascular autonomic failure is associated with upregulated neuroendocrine mechanisms, elevated levels of circulating markers of inflammation that lead to structural and functional cardiac changes and ultimately promote heart failure. In addition to these, prolonged orthostatic stress in patients with OH leads to hyper activation of the endothelin system and activation of compensatory neuroendocrine adaptive mechanisms, eventually the chronic process ends up with a state of "orthostatic hypercoagulation" [47]. Thus, OH promotes atherothrombosis and ischemic events (stroke, coronary artery disease, and myocardial infarction) in the susceptible individuals [8]. According to prospective observational studies, OH is related to mortality, cardiovascular disease events (myocardial infarction and stroke), and incident heart failure [47].

4.2   Conclusion

Although OH prevalence increases with age and comorbidities, it is one key fact that patients admitted to healthcare have been often overlooked.OH not only has close relationship with debilitating diseases such as neurodegenerative diseases, cancer, diabetes, but also carries poor prognosis in itself. OH is a major concern to be overviewed while evaluating especially symptomatic older adults. Therefore, increasing the awareness of clinicians have particular importance.

References

1. Freeman R, Wieling W, Axelrod FB, Benditt DG, Benarroch E, Biaggioni I, et al. Consensus statement on the definition of orthostatic hypotension, neurally mediated syncope and the postural tachycardia syndrome. Clin Auton Res. 2011;21(2):69–72.
2. Brignole M, Moya A, de Lange FJ, Deharo J-C, Elliott PM, Fanciulli A, et al. 2018 ESC Guidelines for the diagnosis and management of syncope. Eur Heart J. 2018;39(21):1883–948.
3. Aydin AE, Soysal P, Isik AT. Which is preferable for orthostatic hypotension diagnosis in older adults: active standing test or head-up tilt table test? Clin Interv Aging. 2017;12:207–12.
4. Mol A, Reijnierse EM, Bui Hoang PTS, van Wezel RJA, Meskers CGM, Maier AB. Orthostatic hypotension and physical functioning in older adults: A systematic review and meta-analysis. Ageing Res Rev. 2018;48:122–44.
5. Isik AT, Kocyigit SE, Smith L, Aydin AE, Soysal P. A comparison of the prevalence of orthostatic hypotension between older patients with Alzheimer's Disease, Lewy body dementia, and without dementia. Exp Gerontol. 2019;124:110628.
6. Chisholm P, Anpalahan M. Orthostatic hypotension: pathophysiology, assessment, treatment and the paradox of supine hypertension. Intern Med J. 2017;47(4):370–9.
7. Duggan E, Romero-Ortuno R, Kenny RA. Admissions for orthostatic hypotension: an analysis of NHS England Hospital Episode Statistics data. BMJ Open. 2019;9(11):e034087.
8. Fedorowski A, Ricci F, Sutton R. Orthostatic hypotension and cardiovascular risk. Kardiol Pol. 2019;77(11):1020–7.
9. Kocyigit SE, Soysal P, Isik AT, Ates Bulut E. Malnutrition and malnutrition risk can be associated with systolic orthostatic hypotension in older adults. J Nutr Health Aging. 2018;22(8):928–33.
10. Kenny RA, Bhangu J. Syncope in older adults. In: Brocklehurst's textbook of geriatric medicine and gerontology. 8th ed. Amsterdam: Elsevier; 2017. p. 335–46.
11. Kocyigit SE, Soysal P, Bulut EA, Aydin AE, Dokuzlar O, Isik AT. What is the relationship between frailty and orthostatic hypotension in older adults? J Geriatr Cardiol. 2019;16(3):272–9.
12. Robertson D. The epidemic of orthostatic tachycardia and orthostatic intolerance. Am J Med Sci. 1999;317(2):75–7.
13. Fedorowski A. ESC CardioMed. In: Orthostatic intolerance: orthostatic hypotension and postural orthostatic tachycardia syndrome. Oxford: Oxford University Press; 2018.
14. Fedorowski A, Melander O. Syndromes of orthostatic intolerance: a hidden danger. J Intern Med. 2013;273(4):322–35.
15. Joseph A, Wanono R, Flamant M, Vidal-Petiot E. Orthostatic hypotension: a review. Nephrol Ther. 2017;13(Suppl 1):S55–s67.
16. Benvenuto LJ, Krakoff LR. Morbidity and mortality of orthostatic hypotension: implications for management of cardiovascular disease. Am J Hypertens. 2011;24(2):135–44.
17. Robertson D, Robertson RM. Causes of chronic orthostatic hypotension. Arch Intern Med. 1994;154(14):1620–4.

18. Shibao C, Grijalva CG, Raj SR, Biaggioni I, Griffin MR. Orthostatic hypotension-related hospitalizations in the United States. Am J Med. 2007;120(11):975–80.
19. Gibbons CH, Schmidt P, Biaggioni I, Frazier-Mills C, Freeman R, Isaacson S, et al. The recommendations of a consensus panel for the screening, diagnosis, and treatment of neurogenic orthostatic hypotension and associated supine hypertension. J Neurol. 2017;264(8):1567–82.
20. McDonell KE, Shibao CA, Claassen DO. Clinical relevance of orthostatic hypotension in neurodegenerative disease. Curr Neurol Neurosci Rep. 2015;15(12):78.
21. Luciano GL, Brennan MJ, Rothberg MB. Postprandial hypotension. Am J Med. 2010;123(3):281.e1–6.
22. Kanjwal K, George A, Figueredo VM, Grubb BP. Orthostatic hypotension: definition, diagnosis and management. J Cardiovasc Med (Hagerstown). 2015;16(2):75–81.
23. Regan CO, Kearney PM, Cronin H, Savva GM, Lawlor BA, Kenny R. Oscillometric measure of blood pressure detects association between orthostatic hypotension and depression in population based study of older adults. BMC Psychiatry. 2013;13:266.
24. Luukinen H, Koski K, Laippala P, Kivela SL. Prognosis of diastolic and systolic orthostatic hypotension in older persons. Arch Intern Med. 1999;159(3):273–80.
25. Rawlings AM, Juraschek SP, Heiss G, Hughes T, Meyer ML, Selvin E, et al. Association of orthostatic hypotension with incident dementia, stroke, and cognitive decline. Neurology. 2018;91(8):e759–e68.
26. Mol A, Bui Hoang PTS, Sharmin S, Reijnierse EM, van Wezel RJA, Meskers CGM, et al. Orthostatic hypotension and falls in older adults: a systematic review and meta-analysis. J Am Med Dir Assoc. 2019;20(5):589–97.e5.
27. Soysal P, Veronese N, Smith L, Torbahn G, Jackson SE, Yang L, et al. Orthostatic hypotension and health outcomes: an umbrella review of observational studies. Eur Geriatr Med. 2019;10(6):863–70.
28. Verwoert GC, Mattace-Raso FU, Hofman A, Heeringa J, Stricker BH, Breteler MM, et al. Orthostatic hypotension and risk of cardiovascular disease in elderly people: the Rotterdam study. J Am Geriatr Soc. 2008;56(10):1816–20.
29. Al-Aama T. Falls in the elderly: spectrum and prevention. Can Fam Physician. 2011;57(7):771–6.
30. Finucane C, O'Connell MD, Donoghue O, Richardson K, Savva GM, Kenny RA. Impaired orthostatic blood pressure recovery is associated with unexplained and injurious falls. J Am Geriatr Soc. 2017;65(3):474–82.
31. Panel on Prevention of Falls in Older Persons, American Geriatrics Society and British Geriatrics Society. Summary of the Updated American Geriatrics Society/British Geriatrics Society clinical practice guideline for prevention of falls in older persons. J Am Geriatr Soc. 2011;59(1):148–57.
32. Sarasin FP, Louis-Simonet M, Carballo D, Slama S, Junod AF, Unger PF. Prevalence of orthostatic hypotension among patients presenting with syncope in the ED. Am J Emerg Med. 2002;20(6):497–501.
33. Ungar A, Mussi C, Ceccofiglio A, Bellelli G, Nicosia F, Bo M, et al. Etiology of Syncope and Unexplained Falls in Elderly Adults with Dementia: Syncope and Dementia (SYD) Study. J Am Geriatr Soc. 2016;64(8):1567–73.
34. Peters R, Anstey KJ, Booth A, Beckett N, Warwick J, Antikainen R, et al. Orthostatic hypotension and symptomatic subclinical orthostatic hypotension increase risk of cognitive impairment: an integrated evidence review and analysis of a large older adult hypertensive cohort. Eur Heart J. 2018;39(33):3135–43.
35. Qiu C, Winblad B, Fratiglioni L. The age-dependent relation of blood pressure to cognitive function and dementia. Lancet Neurol. 2005;4(8):487–99.
36. Sambati L, Calandra-Buonaura G, Poda R, Guaraldi P, Cortelli P. Orthostatic hypotension and cognitive impairment: a dangerous association? Neurol Sci. 2014;35(6):951–7.
37. Rose KM, Couper D, Eigenbrodt ML, Mosley TH, Sharrett AR, Gottesman RF. Orthostatic hypotension and cognitive function: the Atherosclerosis Risk in Communities Study. Neuroepidemiology. 2010;34(1):1–7.

38. Feeney J, O'Leary N, Kenny RA. Impaired orthostatic blood pressure recovery and cognitive performance at two-year follow up in older adults: The Irish Longitudinal Study on Ageing. Clin Auton Res. 2016;26(2):127–33.
39. Andersson M, Hansson O, Minthon L, Ballard CG, Londos E. The period of hypotension following orthostatic challenge is prolonged in dementia with Lewy bodies. Int J Geriatr Psychiatry. 2008;23(2):192–8.
40. Kleipool EEF, Trappenburg MC, Rhodius-Meester HFM, Lemstra AW, van der Flier WM, Peters MJL, et al. Orthostatic hypotension: an important risk factor for clinical progression to mild cognitive impairment or dementia. the amsterdam dementia cohort. J Alzheimers Dis. 2019;71(1):317–25.
41. van Twist DJL, Mostard GJM, Sipers W. Delayed recovery from initial orthostatic hypotension: an expression of frailty in the elderly. Clin Auton Res. 2020;30(2):105–6.
42. Min M, Shi T, Sun C, Liang M, Zhang Y, Bo G, et al. Orthostatic hypotension and the risk of atrial fibrillation and other cardiovascular diseases: An updated meta-analysis of prospective cohort studies. J Clin Hypertens (Greenwich). 2019;21(8):1221–7.
43. Fedorowski A, Burri P, Melander O. Orthostatic hypotension in genetically related hypertensive and normotensive individuals. J Hypertens. 2009;27(5):976–82.
44. SPRINT Research Group, Wright JT Jr, Williamson JD, Whelton PK. A randomized trial of intensive versus standard blood-pressure control. N Engl J Med. 2015;373(22):2103–16.
45. Juraschek SP, Simpson LM, Davis BR, Beach JL, Ishak A, Mukamal KJ. Effects of antihypertensive class on falls, syncope, and orthostatic hypotension in older adults: the allhat trial. Hypertension. 2019;74(4):1033–40.
46. Juraschek SP, Appel LJ, Miller ER 3rd, Mukamal KJ, Lipsitz LA. Hypertension treatment effects on orthostatic hypotension and its relationship with cardiovascular disease. Hypertension. 2018;72(4):986–93.
47. Ricci F, Fedorowski A, Radico F, Romanello M, Tatasciore A, Di Nicola M, et al. Cardiovascular morbidity and mortality related to orthostatic hypotension: a meta-analysis of prospective observational studies. Eur Heart J. 2015;36(25):1609–17.

Diagnosis and Differential Diagnosis

5

Ali Ekrem Aydin and Mehmet Refik Mas

5.1 Introduction

The life expectancy around the world is getting longer, and the population aged 65 and over is growing. Accordingly, the importance of geriatric syndromes becomes more evident. There is a significant decrease in compensatory organ functions that provide homeostatic balance in the body with aging. One of the manifestations that predispose as a result of disruptions in homeostasis is orthostatic hypotension (OH), which can be described as a geriatric syndrome [1].

OH is a common clinical problem that affects 6–30% of community-dwelling older adults, and this rate rises to 60% for inpatients [1, 2]. OH may cause dizziness, blackouts, blurred vision, balance impairment, recurrent falls, dyspnea, angina pectoris, paracervical and lumbar pain, weakness, and nausea [3–5]. However, one-third of elderly adults with OH are asymptomatic [6].

The correct diagnosis of OH in the elderly is of great importance; previous studies demonstrated the association of OH with mortality, ischemic stroke, falls, cognitive failure, impaired sleep quality, depression, renal failure, and cognitive impairment in older adults. Therefore, evaluation of OH should necessarily be a part of the comprehensive geriatric assessment [7–11].

5.2 Diagnosis of OH

In this text, the commonly accepted diagnostic criteria and methods will be explained, as well as different views and approaches in the literature.

A. E. Aydin (✉)
Department of Geriatric Medicine, Sivas State Hospital, Sivas, Turkey

M. R. Mas
International University of Alasia, Nicosia, Cyprus

© Springer Nature Switzerland AG 2021
A. T. Isik, P. Soysal (eds.), *Orthostatic Hypotension in Older Adults*,
https://doi.org/10.1007/978-3-030-62493-4_5

The first description of OH was made in a few cases in 1925; the first consensus criteria were determined in 1996 [12, 13]. According to the consensus statement (CS) on the definition of OH published in 1996, the diagnosis of OH is made in the event of at least 20 mmHg reduction of systolic blood pressure (SBP) and/or at least 10 mmHg reduction of diastolic blood pressure (DBP) within the first 3 min of standing or head-up tilt to at least 60° on a tilt table [13]. The focus of this CS is stated as neurogenic OH (nOH) (OH due to impaired autonomic reflexes results as inadequate sympathetic vasoconstriction). The CS on the definition of OH was updated in 2011, and it was defined as a *sustained* reduction of SBP and/or DBP, and also it would be more appropriate to accept this criterion as a 30 mmHg reduction of SBP in patients with supine hypertension (SH) [14].

The last CS did not mention the time meant by a sustained reduction in BP, but it was shown in a small ($n = 103$) retrospective study that those with who had a sustained (>30 s) BP drop were more likely to have received pharmacological treatment for OH and were more likely to have died in following 5 years than for those has a transient (<30 s) BP drop [15].

In the ESC guideline, a decrease in SBP to <90 mmHg is also specified as a diagnostic criterion for OH, especially in patients with a baseline SBP <110 mmHg [16].

Although there is a consensus report for the diagnosis of OH, discussions about the diagnostic criteria and optimal method continue in the current literature [17–24]: When and how much of blood pressure (BP) drop should be considered? Which approach to perform an orthostatic challenge? Which method to measure BP? Orthostatic symptoms guide the diagnosis or not? Lack of procedural consistency has been emphasized not only in clinical practice but also in studies on OH.

In brief, CS definition on OH is appropriate for screening and standardization in clinical studies, but it should be kept in mind that it may be inadequate for the diagnosis of OH in older adults in clinical practice. The technique, timing, and positioning are the essential variables during an accurate OH evaluation [17–24].

5.3 Variants of OH

The 2011 consensus report also referred to two OH variants, initial and delayed OH [14]:

- **Initial OH (iOH):** A *transient* blood pressure drop (>40 mmHg SBP and/or >20 mmHg diastolic blood pressure) within 15 s of standing [14].

  An active standing test (AST) with continuous blood pressure measurement is preferable to a head-up tilt table test (HUT) to detect iOH more accurately, as beat-to-beat blood pressure monitoring is required [14, 19]. It is thought to be iOH caused by the delay of a reflex response to protect cardiac output after the drop of peripheral vascular resistance rather than autonomic failure [14, 25]. An SBP drop of 20 mmHg and DBP of 10 mmHg should be considered abnormal beyond 30 s after standing up, is seen more frequently with aging [26]. Patients may report that they experience transient orthostatic symptoms as soon as they stand up and improve immediately. The importance of iOH is that it may be one of the underrecognized cause of orthostatic syncope in older adults [25].

- **Delayed OH (dOH)**: OH that develops after the third minute of standing which can be identified with prolonged standing BP, or prolonged HUT. Data about the importance of dOH in the elderly is limited. In a 10-year-follow up study, it has been reported that this phenomenon may be associated with synucleinopathies and mortality. It is thought to be a manifestation of early and less severe autonomic failure [14, 27].

5.4 Screening for OH

Gibbons et al. have grouped patients who should be routinely screened for OH into five categories [28]:

- Patients with suspected or diagnosed neurodegenerative diseases (Parkinson's disease, pure autonomic failure, multiple system atrophy, Lewy body dementia).
- Patients with an unexplained history of falls or syncope.
- Patients with peripheral neuropathies that may be associated with autonomic dysfunction.
- Patients who are elderly (≥ 70 years of age) and frail or who have polypharmacy.
- Patients with orthostatic symptoms.

5.5 Recommendations for Accurate Diagnosis of OH

There are some confounding variables to consider while testing a patient for an accurate diagnosis of OH, like time of the day (diurnal variability), room temperature, food ingestion, state of hydration, medications, age, gender, prolonged recumbency, and deconditioning [14]. Since some of these variables can be optimized, it is stated that it is beneficial to follow some rules while conducting orthostatic tests.

When performing orthostatic tests for diagnosis of OH;

- It should be ensured that the patient does not smoke, take caffeine, or exercise within 30 min before the measurement. (It is known that the mentioned substances can increase BP and exercise can have both BP increasing effect and hypotension effect as stated post-exercise hypotension [29]).
- It should be ensured that measurements are not taken in the postprandial period. (Blood pressure drops may occur within between 15 and 90 s after a meal is known as postprandial hypotension (PPH). It is observed more frequently in the elderly and may be a sign of autonomic failure. PPH develops as a result of inadequate sympathetic compensation to meal-induced splanchnic pooling. It is thought that vasoactive gastrointestinal peptides and insulin also contribute to

vasodilation in the splanchnic circulation, which develops more frequently after large meals, particularly those high in carbohydrates [30].

- To avoid overdiagnoses of OH, auscultatory measurements of BP should be taken by a physician or nurse skilled in the technique recommended by the American Heart Association, with a calibrated manual sphygmomanometer, or a calibrated and automated BP monitor can be preferred for BP measurements [17, 31].

- Patients should be rested in a supine position for 5 min (at least 3 min) in a quiet and 20–24 °C temperature room before the orthostatic test. It is mentioned that there is a little benefit to resting supine longer than 5 min before an orthostatic challenge [32, 33].

5.6   Gray Areas in Timing and Method for Diagnosis of OH

- Since CS on the diagnosis of OH is not described in detail for the optimal timing for BP measurement within 3 min, it may be inadequate for the determination of OH in older adults in clinical practice.

  Measuring BP at different times after standing, before and after 3 min is associated with increased frequency of OH in older adults [18]. Moreover, the diagnosis of OH in clinical practice is time-consuming, which poses difficulties in the evaluation of elderly patients. It is concluded that orthostatic blood pressure changes determined at the first minute may be of higher clinical significance to evaluate OH in elderly patients, compare to the third or fifth minute. A first-minute measurement appears to be adequate for the diagnosis of OH, based on being consistent with the clinical relationships that have been found in the previous studies in clinical practice as it takes a shorter time and identifies most of the cases [23].

  Frith recommended that when using intermittent measurement, evidence supports the first measurement should be taken within the first minute and preferably within the first 30 s, the commonest timing for the BP nadir. It may be considered good practice to measure BP at 60 s intervals with the final measurement at 3 min, according to CS and other studies in the literature [19].

- Although AST and HUT are recommended as methods in CS, there are several studies to evaluate the optimal way for the orthostatic challenge. There is no consensus on the optimum method for diagnosis of OH. Active stand, active sit, sit to stand, squat to stand, and HUT have been evaluated in the previous studies [19, 34–36].

  It still seems to be the most suitable strategy to choose the orthostatic test according to the patient's characteristics in being aware of the advantages and disadvantages of the tests in clinical practice.

  The AST is mentioned in several studies as it has the advantage of reflecting the usual physiological response to standing, and the BP drop is more significant during the AST than HUT. However, many older adults cannot change their positions easily during the transition from supine to the upright position because of existing comorbidities and immobility. An active sitting test or HUT is useful for those who are unable to stand. HUT can help distinguish between nOH and postural tachycardia syndrome (POTS) [37]. (POTS is an exaggerated increase in heart rate as a sustained increment of ≥30 beats/min or ≥120 beats/min heart rate within 10 min of standing or head-up tilt in the absence of OH. It should be noted that this criterion may not be applicable to people with bradycardia. Deconditioning, viral infections, and autonomic disorders are among the causes of POTS [14].)

It is considered that HUT is most useful in documenting objective measures of OH that cannot be obtained in a clinical setting, and it is essential that the evaluation of OH by HUT should be included in daily geriatric practice. European guidelines recommend HUT if the AST is negative, especially if the patient's history suggests OH [17, 38].

- Ambulatory blood pressure monitoring (ABPM) may help confirm the diagnosis of OH in patients with inconsistent BP measurements in the office. When using ABPM for the determination of OH, it should be combined with a posture and orthostatic symptom diary of the patient during monitoring [39]. ABPM also has a valuable role in the diagnosis and monitoring of SH [40].

5.7   Reproducibility

As BP responses to orthostasis are variable because of many confounding factors including diurnal variation, presence of vasoactive hormones, plasma volume, and vasoactive medications, repeated measurements should be done for accurate diagnosis of OH. Probably as a result of these, reproducibility for OH is poor and changes between 57% and 81% [38, 41, 42]. Reproducibility is even weaker in the ward-based setting during a daytime [43]. It has been shown that reproducibility is higher in cases with autonomic failure [42]. OBPC is more severe in the morning, especially when getting out of bed due to prolonged supine position during the night. It might be useful to perform an orthostatic challenge in the morning and try to minimize the confounding factors to improve the reproducibility [37, 42].

5.8   Differential Diagnosis in OH

OH is often classified as neurogenic and non-neurogenic [44]. Another form of classification is acute and chronic OH. Remarkably, the causes of non-neurogenic and acute OH, as well as neurogenic and chronic OH, generally overlap.

Acute OH is usually symptomatic, develops in a short time, and reversible when the underlying cause is resolved. Dehydration, sepsis, adrenal insufficiency, myocardial ischemia, prolonged recumbency or standing, and drugs are examples for acute OH [4, 44].

Chronic OH is usually asymptomatic at baseline, develops over a longer time, and it usually requires pharmacological treatment in addition to non-pharmacological methods. It is often due to autonomic insufficiency secondary to central (dysautonomias, synucleinopathies, brain tumors, brain-stem lesions) or peripheral (diabetes mellitus, dopamine beta-hydroxylase deficiency, paraneoplastic syndrome, vitamin B12 or folate deficiency, alcoholic polyneuropathy, amyloidosis) nervous system diseases [4, 44].

In terms of differential diagnosis, findings on a detailed history and physical examination will be useful for clinical tips for non-neurogenic and neurogenic causes [4, 44].

Findings from laboratory tests and orthostatic tests also will help provide differential diagnosis:

- Physiological response to orthostatic challenge is a small fall in SBP (5–10 mmHg), an increase in DBP (5–10 mmHg), and an increase in pulse rate (10–25 beats per minute) [38].
- An immediate, progressive, and significant decrease in SBP and/or DBP, frequently without an appropriate increase in heart rate, indicates dysautonomia [38].
- An orthostatic drop in BP accompanied by an increase in HR may indicate a nonneurogenic cause, while no increase in HR may indicate nOH [28].
- Neurally mediated (reflex) syncope is characterized by sudden and symptomatic (effects cerebral perfusion) decrease in BP, accompanied by sudden developing bradycardia. Often there are triggering factors such as emotional stress and pain, and prodromal symptoms come first. Postural hemodynamics are normal in these patients, except in acute events. It should be distinguished from syncope due to nOH in patients with chronic autonomic failure. The autonomic response to the Valsalva maneuver is normal, in contrast to autonomic failure [14].
- An exaggerated increase in heart rate as a sustained increment of ≥30 beats/min or ≥120 beats/min heart rate within 10 min of standing or head-up tilt in the absence of OH indicates POTS [14].
- Vertigo is the result of vestibular or cerebellar pathology, but it may be confused with the dizziness or light-headedness of OH. In neurological examination, cerebellar ataxia or nystagmus can be detected, and vestibular testing with electronystagmography shows abnormal responses [45].
- OH, should be evaluated in a patient who applied to the clinic due to a fall. On the other hand, falls due to other causes in the elderly should be questioned. Falling due to sensory disorders and orthopedic problems can be given as examples. Discrimination can be provided with a detailed history and physical examination. Neurologic examination may show gait imbalance or abnormal postural reflexes [46].
- Psychogenic pseudo-syncope is characterized by periods of unresponsiveness due to psychiatric disorders. It could be confused with syncope. A psychiatric evaluation may be helpful in determining the cause. Normal HUT responses may be suggestive for the diagnosis [16].

5.9   Conclusions

Correct evaluation of orthostatic hypotension (OH) is crucial in geriatric practice since OH is associated with mortality and morbidity. It is important to evaluate the patient for OH, even if it is asymptomatic, considering the increased frequency of OH in the elderly. CS on the definition of OH that made in 2011 is appropriate for screening and standardization OH in clinical studies, but it should be kept in mind that it may be inadequate for the diagnosis of OH in older adults in clinical practice. It may be favorable to perform OH evaluation at each visit, considering the low reproducibility of OH.

References

1. Feldstein C, Weder AB. Orthostatic hypotension: a common, serious and underrecognized problem in hospitalized patients. J Am Soc Hypertens. 2012;6(1):27–39. https://doi.org/10.1016/j.jash.2011.08.008.
2. Chen S-Y, Chen CH, Chang CM. Management of orthostatic hypotension in the elderly. J Nurs. 2010;57(5):89–95.
3. Fedorowski A, Melander O. Syndromes of orthostatic intolerance: a hidden danger. J Intern Med. 2013;273(4):322–35.
4. Gupta V, Lipsitz LA. Orthostatic hypotension in the elderly: diagnosis and treatment. Am J Med. 2007;120(10):841–7.
5. Shibao C, Lipsitz LA, Biaggioni I. Evaluation and treatment of orthostatic hypotension. J Am Soc Hypertens. 2013;7(4):317–24.
6. Arbogast SD, Alshekhlee A, Hussain Z, McNeeley K, Chelimsky TC. Hypotension unawareness in profound orthostatic hypotension. Am J Med. 2009;122(6):574–80.
7. Galizia G, Convertino G, Testa G, Langellotto A, Rengo F, Abete P. Transient ischemic attack caused by delayed orthostatic hypotension in an elderly hypertensive patient. Geriatr Gerontol Int. 2012;12:565–7.
8. Gangavati A, Hajjar I, Quach L, Jones RN, Kiely DK, Gagnon P, et al. Hypertension, orthostatic hypotension, and the risk of falls in a community-dwelling elderly population: the maintenance of balance, independent living, intellect, and zest in the elderly of Boston study. J Am Geriatr Soc. 2011;59(3):383–9.
9. Mehrabian S, Duron E, Labouree F, Rollot F, Bune A, Traykov L, et al. Relationship between orthostatic hypotension and cognitive impairment in the elderly. J Neurol Sci. 2010;299(1–2):45–8.
10. McHugh JE, Fan CW, Kenny RA, Lawlor BA. Orthostatic hypotension and subjective sleep quality in older people. Aging Ment Heal. 2012;16(8):958–63. http://www.tandfonline.com/doi/pdf/10.1080/13607863.2012.684665
11. Soysal P, Yay A, Isik AT. Does vitamin D deficiency increase orthostatic hypotension risk in the elderly patients? Arch Gerontol Geriatr. 2014;59(1):74–7.
12. Bradbury S, Eggleston C. Postural hypotension. A report of three cases. Am Heart J. 1925;1:73–86.
13. Consensus statement on the definition of orthostatic hypotension, pure autonomic failure, and multiple system atrophy. The consensus Committee of the American Autonomic Society and the American Academy of Neurology. Neurology. 1996;46(5):1470.
14. Freeman R, Wieling W, Axelrod FB, Benditt DG, Benarroch E, Biaggioni I, et al. Consensus statement on the definition of orthostatic hypotension, neurally mediated syncope and the postural tachycardia syndrome. Clin Auton Res. 2011;21(2):69–72.

15. Frith J, Bashir AS, Newton JL. The duration of the orthostatic blood pressure drop is predictive of death. QJM. 2016;109(4):231–5.
16. Brignole M, Moya A, de Lange FJ, Deharo J-C, Elliott PM, Fanciulli A, et al. ESC guidelines for the diagnosis and management of syncope. Eur Heart J. 2018;39(21):1883–948.
17. Aydin AE, Soysal P, Isik AT. Which is preferable for orthostatic hypotension diagnosis in older adults: active standing test or head-up tilt table test? Clin Interv Aging. 2017;12:207–12.
18. Campos ACR, de Almeida NA, Ramos AL, Vasconcelos DF, Freitas MP, de V Toledo MA. Orthostatic hypotension at different times after standing erect in elderly adults. J Am Geriatr Soc. 2015;63:589–90.
19. Frith J. Diagnosing orthostatic hypotension: a narrative review of the evidence. Br Med Bull. 2015;115(1):123–34.
20. Grubb BP, Kosinski DJ. Syncope resulting from autonomic insufficiency syndromes associated with orthostatic intolerance. Med Clin North Am. 2001;85(2):457–72.
21. Juraschek SP, Daya N, Rawlings AM, Appel LJ, Miller ER 3rd, Windham BG, et al. Association of History of dizziness and long-term adverse outcomes with early vs. later orthostatic hypotension assessment times in middle-aged adults. JAMA Intern Med. 2017;177(9):1316–23.
22. Kunert MP. Evaluation and management of orthostatic hypotension in elderly individuals. J Gerontol Nurs. 1999;25(3):42–6.
23. Soysal P, Aydin AE, Koc Okudur S, Isik AT. When should orthostatic blood pressure changes be evaluated in elderly: 1st, 3rd or 5th minute? Arch Gerontol Geriatr. 2016;65:199–203.
24. Cheshire WPJ. Clinical classification of orthostatic hypotensions. Clin Auton Res. 2017;27:133–5.
25. Wieling W, Krediet CTP, van Dijk N, Linzer M, Tschakovsky ME. Initial orthostatic hypotension: review of a forgotten condition. Clin Sci (Lond). 2007;112(3):157–65.
26. Finucane C, O'Connell MDL, Fan CW, Savva GM, Soraghan CJ, Nolan H, et al. Age-related normative changes in phasic orthostatic blood pressure in a large population study: findings from the Irish longitudinal study on ageing (TILDA). Circulation. 2014;130(20):1780–9.
27. Gibbons CH, Freeman R. Delayed orthostatic hypotension: a frequent cause of orthostatic intolerance. Neurology. 2006;67(1):28–32.
28. Gibbons CH, Schmidt P, Biaggioni I, Frazier-Mills C, Freeman R, Isaacson S, et al. The recommendations of a consensus panel for the screening, diagnosis, and treatment of neurogenic orthostatic hypotension and associated supine hypertension. J Neurol. 2017;264(8):1567–82.
29. Santaella DF, Araújo EA, Ortega KC, Tinucci T, Mion DJ, Negrão CE, et al. Aftereffects of exercise and relaxation on blood pressure. Clin J Sport Med. 2006;16(4):341–7.
30. Jansen RW, Lipsitz LA. Postprandial hypotension: epidemiology, pathophysiology, and clinical management. Ann Intern Med. 1995;122(0003–4819 (Print)):286–95. c:%5CEMH%5CScannede artikler referanser%5CRefMan6528.pdf
31. Curb JD, Labarthe DR, Cooper SP, Cutter GR, Hawkins CM. Training and certification of blood pressure observers. Hypertension. 1983;5(4):610–4.
32. Frith J, Reeve P, Newton JL. Length of time required to achieve a stable baseline blood pressure in the diagnosis of orthostatic hypotension. J Am Geriatr Soc. 2013;61:1414–5.
33. Lahrmann H, Cortelli P, Hilz M, Mathias CJ, Struhal W, Tassinari M. EFNS guidelines on the diagnosis and management of orthostatic hypotension. Eur J Neurol. 2006;13(9):930–6.
34. Cooke J, Carew S, Quinn C, O'Connor M, Curtin J, O'Connor C, et al. The prevalence and pathological correlates of orthostatic hypotension and its subtypes when measured using beat-to-beat technology in a sample of older adults living in the community. Age Ageing. 2013;42(6):709–14.
35. Cohen N, Gorelik O, Fishlev G, Almoznino-Sarafian D, Alon I, Shteinshnaider M, et al. Seated postural hypotension is common among older inpatients. Clin Auton Res. 2003;13(6):447–9.
36. Rossberg F, Penaz J. Initial cardiovascular response on change of posture from squatting to standing. Eur J Appl Physiol Occup Physiol. 1988;57(1):93–7.
37. Low PA, Tomalia VA, Park K-J. Autonomic function tests: some clinical applications. J Clin Neurol. 2013;9(1):1–8.

38. Lamarre-Cliche M, Cusson J. The fainting patient: value of the head-upright tilt-table test in adult patients with orthostatic intolerance. CMAJ. 2001;164(3):372–6.
39. Norcliffe-Kaufmann L, Kaufmann H. Is ambulatory blood pressure monitoring useful in patients with chronic autonomic failure? Clin Auton Res. 2014;24(4):189–92.
40. Pickering TG, Shimbo D, Haas D. Ambulatory blood-pressure monitoring. N Engl J Med. 2006;354(22):2368–74.
41. Naschitz JE, Rosner I. Orthostatic hypotension: framework of the syndrome. Postgrad Med J. 2007;83(983):568–74.
42. Ward C, Kenny RA. Reproducibility of orthostatic hypotension in symptomatic elderly. Am J Med. 1996;100(4):418–22.
43. Belmin J, Abderrhamane M, Medjahed S, Sibony-Prat J, Bruhat A, Bojic N, et al. Variability of blood pressure response to orthostatism and reproducibility of the diagnosis of orthostatic hypotension in elderly subjects. J Gerontol A Biol Sci Med Sci. 2000;55(11):M667–71.
44. Mathias CJ. Orthostatic hypotension: causes, mechanisms, and influencing factors. Neurology. 1995;45(4 Suppl 5):S6–11.
45. Swain SK, Anand N, Mishra S. Vertigo among elderly people: current opinion. J Med Soc. 2019;33(1):1–5;
46. Ooi WL, Hossain M, Lipsitz LA. The association between orthostatic hypotension and recurrent falls in nursing home residents. Am J Med. 2000;108(2):106–11.

Orthostatic Hypotension and Drugs: Drug-Induced Orthostatic Hypotension

6

Suha Beril Kadioglu and Turgay Celik

Abbreviations

ACE	Angiotensin Converting Enzyme
CCBs	Calcium Channel blockers
DOH	Drug-Induced Orthostatic Hypotension
L-DOPA	Levodopa
OH	Orthostatic Hypotension
PD	Parkinson's Disease
TCAs	Tricyclic Antidepressants

6.1 Introduction

Drug-Induced Orthostatic Hypotension (DOH) is an unnoticeable finding or symptom and one of secondary OHs in the elderly [1]. DOH or symptoms are associated with increased neurodegenerative changes or diseases leading to autonomic nervous system (ANS) malfunctioning. If DOH is not asymptomatic, DOH like OH is usually manifested by varying degrees of light-headedness on standing, a symptom tolerated by most individuals. In more progressive periods, it is inevitable that it leads to syncope, falls, injury, cerebrovascular accidents, and myocardial infarction as a result of reduced perfusion. Normally, decreased blood pressure is prevented by autonomy tone or reflex sympathetic system activation with an increase in heart rate, and constriction of peripheral veins and arteries, but not works sufficiently in patients with OH. Therefore, impairment or dysfunction of autonomic tone (or

S. B. Kadioglu · T. Celik (✉)
Department of Pharmacology, Faculty of Pharmacy, Yeditepe University of Medical Sciences, İstanbul, Turkey
e-mail: turgay.celik@yeditepe.edu.tr

© Springer Nature Switzerland AG 2021
A. T. Isik, P. Soysal (eds.), *Orthostatic Hypotension in Older Adults*,
https://doi.org/10.1007/978-3-030-62493-4_6

reflexes) that regulate blood pressure may lead to OH. DOH is frequent due to drugs that may interfere with autonomic function (e.g., antihypertensive drugs, antidepressants, diuretics, and blocker drugs for the treatment of urinary retention), diseases which causes peripheral autonomic neuropathies such as diabetes, and less widely, primary degenerative disorders of the ANS [2]. As a result, orthostatic hypotension may be frequently triggered or developed easily by drugs in elderly and DOH occurs. The presence of DOH reflects a functional or structural sympathetic denervation or a deranged reflex readjustment of sympathetic outflow DOH frequently observed in elderly and patients with neurodegenerative diseases, diabetes, or hypertension.

In 1996, OH was described, as a drop in systolic blood pressure ≥ 20 mmHg or diastolic blood pressure ≥ 10 mmHg on postural challenge, with or without symptoms, after 3 min of standing or head-up tilt to at least 60° on a tilt table, by the American Academy of Neurology and the American Autonomic Society. In 2011, the definition was updated, as initial and delayed OH. A transient blood pressure decline (≥ 40 mmHg systolic blood pressure and/or ≥ 20 mmHg diastolic blood pressure) within 15 s of standing is defined as initial OH, whereas OH that occurs beyond 3 min of postural challenge, was defined as delayed OH [2]. Position change from supine to the upright is the significant parameter responsible for the degree of the decrease. Also, the occurrence of the symptoms of OH is due to the degree of decrease, rather than the low blood pressure value [3].

6.2 Epidemiology

OH is very common, affecting one in five community-dwelling older people, the prevalence ranges from 5% to 30%, increases with age and mostly seen in patients ≥ 65 years old [4–6]. Prevalence studies indicating that about 25% of type II diabetic patients, 30% of people aged ≥ 65 years, and 70% of Parkinson's disease patients are experiencing orthostatic hypotension [7]. Symptoms of patients suffering from OH are light-headedness, dizziness, nausea, weakness or blurred vision during in standing position. Due to the nonspecific symptoms of orthostatic hypotension like dizziness, fatigue, difficulties in concentration, and vision problems, it is estimated that it is a more common issue among geriatric population [8]. Risk factors are medications (particularly antihypertensive drugs), smoking, being on a bed rest for a long time and some comorbidities. Initial period of neurodegenerative diseases including Parkinson's disease and neuropathic diseases like Diabetes mellitus may provoke DOH, which is closely related to instability of autonomic nervous system, but it is also a frequent symptom among hypertensive patients [9] and frailty in elderly patients [10]. On the other hand, the underlying cause of the non-neurogenic OH may be hypovolemia, which can be caused by disorders such as chronic bleeding, diabetes insipidus, adrenal insufficiency, diarrhea or dehydration [3, 5, 11].

Increased diurnal BP variabilities and hypertension, which are both present in cases of primary and secondary OH, may provoke episodic attacks with increased afterload, leading to permanent organ damage, such as left ventricular hypertrophy and reduced renal function, high risk of congestive heart failure, and also ischemia in myocardium. Moreover, altered autonomic tone in patients with hypertension [13] and sleep apnea [12]is known to be associated with the development of atrial fibrillation [14], which is itself accepted as a famous risk factor for heart failure [13, 14].

Disruption of blood pressure homeostasis is account for increasing the actions of neuroendocrine compensatory systems, also will possibly promote the occurrence of cardiovascular or cerebrovascular events. Supporting this theory, vascular endothelin system hyperactivation has been detected in patients with fall or syncope due to OH [15]. Therefore, endothelin 1 and vasopressin, which are considered as endogen vasoconstrictors and play a role to maintain adaptive mechanisms along orthostatic hypotensive stress, may cause atherothrombotic vascular events in predisposed individuals [16]. However, current literatures do not display us until now to reach any conclusion as to whether OH is a sign of mortality risk, an intermediate variable of the cardiovascular risk factors, a stage of disease severity, or a different causative mechanism.

6.3 Drug-Induced Orthostatic Hypotension

Patients with DOH may show abnormal responses to a lot of pharmacological conditions or physiological changes, such as wide fluctuations in BP [17]. Medications and diseases conditions that may produce functional disruption of the autonomic nervous system cover treatment with antihypertensive drugs (vasodilators, α-adrenergic receptor antagonists, calcium channel blockers, diuretics, angiotensin converting enzyme inhibitors, diuretics, and β-adrenergic receptor blockers) antidepressants, antipsychotics and chemotherapeutic agents; relative decrease in circulating volume; peripheral venous pooling; and congestive heart failure [18]. List of drug groups causing OH are shown in Table 6.1.

Although, DOH is seen in patients who have progressive changes in cardiovascular physiology associated with normal aging, most patients do not experience OH unless they have concurrent diseases, or the patient is receiving drugs which are known to induce hypotension. There are increased number of unrecognized cases as majority of patients with OH are having few nonspecific findings and they are usually asymptomatic.

OH Patients may also suffer from wide BP swings and also recumbent hypertension, or they may have abnormal responses to some pharmacological or physiological difficulties [17, 19].

Immobilization, alcohol drinking, alcohol drinking, post-exercise, heat and fever are considered as predisposing conditions to dehydration and venous pooling, which may exacerbate the symptoms especially in the mornings after waking up. After consumption of large meals with carbohydrate-rich food, patients with autonomic dysfunction become more open to occurrence of postprandial hypotension, as a result of gastric distension, release of vasodilator endogen peptides and splanchnic blood pooling [20]. Nocturnal polyuria, resulting from the distribution of peripheral

Table 6.1 Main drug groups causing orthostatic hypotension

Calcium Channel blockers
Vasodilators (nitrates)
Angiotensin converting enzyme inhibitors
Diuretics
α-Adrenergic receptor antagonists
β-Adrenergic receptor blockers
Sympatholytics
Antipsychotics
Antianginals
Antiarrhythmics
Anti-parkinsonian drugs
Antidepressants
Monoamine oxidase inhibitors
Dopamine receptor agonists
Drugs for erectile dysfunction
Chemotherapeutic agents
Phenothiazines
Narcotics/tranquilizers/sedatives

Table 6.2 Predisposing factors affecting orthostatic hypotension by normal aging [28]

Predisposing factors		
Vascular	Cardiac	Renal
• Decreased baroreceptor activity • Decreased arterial compliance • Increased venous capacity • Decreased plasma volume • Low cerebral blood flow • Decrease in vasopressin response (via V_1 receptors)	• Reduced cardiac compliance • Reduced cardiac output	• Reduced renin/angiotensin activity • Decrease in vasopressin response (via V_2 receptors) • Reduced renal sodium conservation

blood to central regions in supine status, is a common complaint and also aggravated by natriuresis with accompanying supine hypertension. Thereby, tendency to morning hypotension may be enhanced in these patients and they may suffer from decreased intravascular volume overnight.

6.4 The Relationship of Orthostatic Hypotension with Age

Most patients with DOH are asymptomatic or have few nonspecific symptoms, so, it is very hard to predict the rate of unrecognized cases [21]. However, aging is the most important risk factor for DOH like OH [22, 23], also with some medications (nitrates, antihypertensive drugs, α-adrenergic blockers, antidepressants, polypharmacy) [24, 25] and other unspecific factors worsening OH (alcoholism, female sex, increased body temperature, insufficient body mass index, and smoking [26, 27]. Predisposing and protective factors affecting OH by normal aging are shown in Table 6.2 [28]. When the central arterial pressure and cerebral perfusion related with cerebral tissue oxygenation declines critically during OH, patients may additionally report dizziness, blurred vision, fatigue, and, finally, suffer from loss of consciousness.

In the early periods of aging, low blood pressure or OH symptoms are not always observed with DOH, but may be triggered by medications. When there is an increase in neurodegenerative changes, OH symptoms including dizziness, light-headedness, and syncope, all related to insufficient blood flow to brain regions, and also fatigue, weakness, blurred vision, hearing impairments or cognitive slowing may be observed [21, 29]. As known, DOH is usually asymptomatic [21], but carries a risk for falls, syncope or cognitive dysfunction like OH [7]. If patients with DOH have symptoms at young and middle-ages, various neurodegenerative diseases are manifested by OH and it can be seen in early stages of the disease by some drugs. However, autonomic dysfunction is low to be drug-triggered or the level of disruption in the autonomic neuron is not enough [22].

6.5 Pathophysiology

Pathologically, OH are often classified as primary and secondary types [30] and clinically are subdivided into acute and chronic forms [17]. DOH, is considered as a secondary OH, it is triggered by medications and some chronic diseases such as diabetes mellitus and cardiovascular diseases. OH can be classified into pathophysiological categories as neurogenic (structural) and non-neurogenic (functional) causes of autonomic dysfunctions. Neurogenic OH is a critical manifestation of autonomic dysfunction related with primary chronic neurodegenerative disorders, such as multiple system atrophy, or Parkinson disease, however the diseases that cause neurological disorders such as diabetes, polypharmacy, or advanced renal failure can cause secondary type [30, 31].OH resulting from the autonomic dysfunctions originated to a primary neurodegenerative disease, is usually considered as neurogenic OH. Some systemic illnesses producing peripheral neuropathy can cause secondary autonomic dysfunction or failure. The etiology of secondary OH leading to autonomic dysfunctions is shown in Table 6.3.

Dysautonomic manifestations related with neurodegenerative changes cause OH by the relation of different parts of the autonomous nervous system in elderly. For example, autonomic dysfunction of the cardiovascular system is connected to a loss or decrease of peripheral noradrenergic innervation. All of these dysautonomic symptoms are mainly associated to preganglionic autonomic neuron degeneration of the brainstem and spinal cord [32]. Although, there are many different symptom-specific scales that clinically being used, they are insufficient to identify OH symptoms according to degree of neuropathology or aging and to estimate OH prevalence [33].

Table 6.3 Etiology of autonomic dysfunction related with secondary orthostatic hypotension

Polypharmacy
Iatrogenic (drug-related)
Older age
Diabetes mellitus
Cerebrovascular disease
Cardiovascular diseases (essential hypertension, pulmonary hypertension, sick-sinus syndrome, AV-block, heart failure, aortic stenosis)
Renal failure
Volume reduction
Venous pooling
Polyneuropathy (alcohol and other)
Endocrine disorders (diabetes insipidus, adrenal insufficiency, thyroid diseases)
Amyloidosis
Autoimmune diseases
Multiple myeloma
Paraneoplastic syndromes
Multiple sclerosis
Spinal cord diseases

6.6   The Control Mechanisms in Maintaining Blood Pressure

Regulation mechanisms of BP are complicated physiological functions depending on continuous actions of the cardiovascular, endocrine renal and neurologic systems [31]. While central blood flow maintains as control of BP through the changes in vascular tonus and cardiac output, regional blood flow occurs through local mediators (eicosanoids, endothelin, nitric oxide, and tissue plasminogen activators). The maintenance of these physiological changes is provided by the intact autonomic nervous system consisting of the parasympathetic and sympathetic nervous systems. The sympathetic nervous system determines the size or magnitude of arterial BP and the distribution and regulation of cardiac output [32]. Therefore, adrenergic receptors will be discussed extensively in below. The parasympathetic contribution to the setting of vascular tone is less importance.

Baroreceptors and chemoreceptor feedback reflex mechanisms regulate the short-term reflex control of the sympathetic vasomotor activities. In cases of different external stimuli or stresses, central mechanisms will also produce sympathetic activities [33]. The long term control of cardiovascular homeostasis depends on various mechanisms, including renal changes in the control of extracellular volume, natriuresis, the levels of sympathetic vasomotor activity, and the renin-angiotensin-aldosterone systems [33–35].

DOH can be well accomplished by solving the likely causes and understanding the mechanisms related with the maintenance of blood pressure due to sudden position changes. Considering the effect of gravity, standing up causes the translocation of blood to lower parts of the body, decreased venous return and eventually reduced stroke volume and decreased cardiac output [5]. Compensating actions of the body

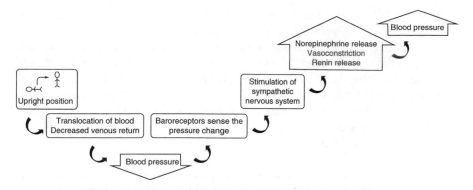

Fig. 6.1 Compensating actions to regulate blood pressure in response to standing

includes (1) muscle pump, (2) baroreflex mechanisms and (3) renin-angiotensin-aldosterone system (Fig. 6.1):

1. In the upright position, approximately 600 ml of blood are redistributed and pooled in lower extremities, venous return of the circulating blood to the heart is decreased. Muscle contractions compress capacitance vessels, increase venous return, and inhibit the excess pooling of the blood in lower parts of the body. Skeletal and gluteal muscles pump blood from the legs and force blood supply to the heart through the venous system. These muscle contractions are considered as the primary defense against decreased venous return [5, 36, 37].

2. The neurovascular adjustments start with a decrease in blood pressure and this decrease is detected immediately by the baroreceptors. These baroreceptors which are responsible from sensing the pressure changes, are located in the carotid sinus, intima of the aortic arch and also in the walls of the atrium and ventricles. When there is a sudden decrease in blood pressure, this information is noticed by baroreceptors, integrated in the medulla and the compensatory mechanisms are stimulated. This mechanism in the heart and vessels works within seconds via sympathetic nervous system. Increased norepinephrine release and α-adrenergic receptor stimulation lead to vasoconstriction and causes blood to move toward the upper parts of the body. Standing up causes a temporary drop in afferent arteriole perfusion pressure. Low or decrease in renal arterial pressure and sympathetic neural activity (through β-adrenergic receptors) stimulates release of renin by the juxtaglomerular apparatus and triggers the renin-angiotensin-aldosterone system [5, 36, 37].

3. Renin-angiotensin-aldosterone system is a longer-lasting control mechanism for the regulation of blood pressure. Angiotensinogen, which is produced in the liver, is converted to angiotensin I by an enzyme called renin. Renin production increases in case of reduction in sodium levels and in blood pressure, which is perceived by the kidneys. Decreased blood pressure can stimulate the sympa-

thetic activity, and also renin secretion is increased via β_1-adrenergic receptors. Angiotensin I, an important active precursor, is cleaved by the angiotensin converting enzyme to produce angiotensin II. Angiotensin II, a more active form leads to direct constriction of resistance vessels and stimulates the secretion of aldosterone from the adrenal glands. Aldosterone increases renal reabsorption of sodium and therefore leads to elevated blood sodium and increasing water retention and blood volume. These homeostatic actions of the renin–angiotensin aldosterone system occurs in minutes and hours, and responsible from the regulation of blood pressure [5, 36, 38].

6.7   Drug-Mediated Dysfunctions of Blood Pressure Maintenance in Older Age

The compensating actions of the body may become insufficient as a result of some age-related structural changes. Especially, evaluation of age-related pathological changes in the vessels should be the starting point of orthostatic hypotension. Advanced age may promote pathophysiological modifications that result in ineffective compensation to blood pressure changes. These modifications include thickening and dilation of large arteries, increased stiffness of barosensory vessel walls and decreased effectiveness of cardio-vagal autonomic control [39, 40]. Venous pooling and decreased venous return cause a reduced stroke volume due to the change of supine to standing position, and therefore decreases cardiac output. The natural response of the cardiovascular system will be increasing the heart rate and vasoconstriction in order to maintain blood supply to the cerebral tissues. In the elderly, blood vessels become inadequate to respond these blood pressure changes, and heart rate is more stable. These alterations of the autonomic nervous system have an important role in the development of age-dependent increase of the prevalence of OH [41]. On the other hand, the blood volume is reduced owing to the dehydration or reduced hematopoiesis in geriatric patients. These age-related changes that contribute to the occurrence of OH, are not temporary and will deteriorate consistently over time [42]. Risk of OH is increasing not only because of the pathophysiological changes but also some medical interventions, considering the fact that geriatric patients are under treatment with medications (prescription and non-prescription drugs) that may attenuate the normal physiologic response to standing. Also, regarding the increased prevalence of polypharmacy in elderly patients, DOH should become under review [19].

OH is a side effect of many common medications used by older persons including for α-adrenergic receptor antagonists, calcium channel blockers, diuretics, angiotensin converting enzyme inhibitors, antipsychotics, beta-adrenergic receptor blockers, anti-Parkinsonian drugs, antianginal, and antidepressant medications [24, 28]. All of the drugs that could potentially cause OH side effects are presented on Table 6.4 [43]. However, the drugs leading to potentially If OH occurrence is a side effects of drug, it need to evaluate again potential predisposing factors for definition of pathology. In some cases, it may be difficult and hazardous to stop the offending

Table 6.4   List of the drugs that lead to orthostatic hypotension and hypotension as side effect [43]

Drugs with orthostatic hypotension side effects				
Irinotecan	Labetalol	Pramipexole	Tamsulosin	
Drugs with hypotension side effects				
Acamprosate	Clonidine	Imipramine	Olanzapine	Silodosin
Acebutolol	Clozapine	Indapamide	Olmesartan	Sitagliptin
Alfuzosin	Codeine	Irbesartan	Olsalazine	Sitaxsentan
Amantadine	Conivaptan	Irinotecan	Oxcarbazepine	Sodium nitroprusside
Amiloride	Dacarbazine	Isocarboxazid	Oxprenolol	Sparfloxacin
Amisulpride	Dapagliflozin	Isosorbide	Oxycodone	Tacrolimus
Amitriptyline	Delavirdine	Itraconazole	Oxymorphone	Tadalafil
Amlodipine	Deprenyl	Ivermectin	Paclitaxel	Tamsulosin
Amphotericin B	Desmopressin	Ketoconazole	Paliperidone	Telmisartan
Anagrelide	Desvenlafaxine	Labetalol	Parecoxib	Terazosin
Apomorphine	Diazepam	Lamotrigine	Paroxetine	Tetrabenazine
Aripiprazole	Diltiazem	Lercanidipine	Pergolide	Thalidomide
Asenapine	Dipyridamole	Leuprorelin	Perindopril	Thiazide
Atenolol	Docetaxel	Levodopa	Perphenazine	Tiagabine
Atorvastatin	Dolasetron	Levomepromazine	Phenelzine	Tizanidine
Azilsartan	Donepezil	Linaclotide	Phenoxybenzamine	Tolvaptan
Baclofen	Dothiepin	Lisuride	Phentolamine	Topiramate
Benazepril	Doxazosin	Losartan	Phenylephrine	Tramadol
Bendrofluazide	Doxorubicin	Loxapine	Phenytoin	Trazodone
Betahistine	Duloxetine	Lurasidone	Pimozide	Trospium chloride
Bisoprolol	Empagliflozin	Maprotiline	Pindolol	Valproate
Bortezomib	Entacapone	Maraviroc	Polythiazide	Valsartan
Bosentan	Eplerenone	Mecamylamine	Posaconazole	Vardenafil
Bretylium	Eprosartan	Medroxyprogesterone	Pramipexole	Venlafaxine
Bromocriptine	Eslicarbazepine	Memantine	Prazosin	Verapamil
Bupivacaine	Ethionamide	Meperidine	Pregabalin	Vinflunine
Buprenorphine	Etoricoxib	Methadone	Propafenone	Voriconazole
Bupropion	Felodipine	Methysergide	Prostacyclin	Zaleplon
Cabazitaxel	Fenoldopam	Metolazone	Protriptyline	Ziconotide
Cabergoline	Fentanyl	Metoprolol	Quetiapine	Ziprasidone
Canagliflozin	Finasteride	Mirtazapine	Quinapril	Zolmitriptan
Candesartan	Flunitrazepam	Mitotane	Quinaprilat	Zolpidem
Capecitabine	Fluoxetine	Moexiprilat	Quinidine	
Captopril	Fluvoxamine	Morphine	Ramipril	
Carbamazepine	Fosinopril	Moxifloxacin	Ranolazine	
Carbidopa	Fosphenytoin	Moxonidine	Rapamycin	
Carisoprodol	Furosemide	Mycophenolate	Rasagiline	
Carvedilol	Gadobutrol	Mycophenolic acid	Reboxetine	
Cevimeline	Galantamine	Nabilone	Rifapentine	
Chlorpromazine	Granisetron	Nefazodone	Riluzole	
Chlorthalidone	Guanfacine	Niacin	Risperidone	
Cidofovir	Halofantrine	Nicardipine	Ritonavir	
Cilazapril	Haloperidol	Nicorandil	Rivastigmine	
Cilostazol	Hydrochlorothiazide	Nifedipine	Ropinirole	
Ciprofloxacin	Hydroflumethiazide	Nisoldipine	Ropivacaine	
Cisplatin	Hydromorphone	Nitroglycerin	Rotigotine	
Citalopram	Ibutilide	Norfloxacin	Sertraline	
Clomipramine	Icodextrin	Nortriptyline	Sibutramine	
Clonazepam	Iloperidone	Ofloxacin	Sildenafil	

medications. In these cases, different treatment strategies including the use of salt tablets, elevation of the head of the bed, and fludrocortisone administration may be instituted prior to or while continuing the offending medication [44]. However, the main strategy in DOH is to change the treatment of the disease that causes drug use and then to confirm it.

6.8   α-Adrenergic Receptor Antagonists

Antihypertensive mechanism of action ofα-adrenergic receptor antagonists is the selective blockade of postsynaptic α_1 receptors located both in arterioles and venules. This blockade results a decrease in arterial blood pressure because of dilation in both resistance and capacitance vessels. Therefore, patients under therapy with α_1 receptor blockers are likely to have decreased blood pressure when changing from supine position to the upright position. Monitorization of the blood pressure should be maintained especially for elderly patients [28, 36, 45].α_2 receptor stimulation in the brain results in presynaptic inhibition or in a decrease in the release of norepinephrine from the vasomotor center centrally, increases the vagal tone and therefore reduces the blood pressure. The decrease in sympathetic tonus may result in decreased heart rate, cardiac output, peripheral resistance, level of plasma renin and activity of baroreceptor reflexes, therefore, may cause OH.

6.9   Diuretics

Diuretics are effective in lowering blood pressure by depleting the sodium stores in the great majority of patients and thereby causing volume depletion by increasing the volume of urine excreted. The decrease in plasma volume that results in response to an increased urine and Na excretion, lowers cardiac output and venous return. Most side effects of diuretics are, generally dose-dependent, including hyponatremia, hypovolemia, and hypotension. Diuretics can be used as monotherapy in patients with mild to moderate primary hypertension. In patients with severe hypertension, diuretics can be used in combination with sympatholytic and vasodilator drugs. Also, in the elderly, when considering the dehydration, weakness and volume depletion in these patients, the risk of OH due to the diuretic therapy will be increased [28, 36, 46, 47].

6.10   Angiotensin Converting Enzyme (ACE) Inhibitors

ACE Inhibitors inhibit competitively the activity of ACE (alşo termed kininase II) to prevent formation of angiotensin II (more active octapeptide) from angiotensin I (less active decapeptide). Its reduce total peripheral resistance and systolic and diastolic BP by decreasing vasoconstrictor effects of angiotensin II and sodium-retaining activities through aldosterone. ACE is also named as plasma kininase, which is responsible from the breakdown of a potent vasodilator bradykinin. Therefore, ACE inhibitors increase the actions of the kallikrein—kinin system, and the release of nitric oxide and prostacyclin will be increased. Patients with low cardiac output like in congestive heart failure and also patients with high plasma renin activity may experience excessive fall in blood pressure and are at risk of OH [28, 42, 47, 48].

6.11 Calcium Channel Blockers

Calcium channel blockers (CCBs) act on the L-type calcium channels found in the vascular smooth muscle and cardiac myocytes. Blockade of these channels inhibits the influx of calcium into muscle cells, thereby results in the inhibition of smooth muscle contraction and also cardiac muscle contraction [49].Dihydropyridine calcium channel blockers inhibit calcium influx into arterial smooth muscle cells and cause vasodilation more selectively, and their depressant effect on the heart is less than verapamil and diltiazem. Dihydropyridine calcium channel blockers require monitoring in elderly patients with hypertension, as they are potent vasodilators and overdose can lead to an excessive fall in blood pressure, also postural hypotension [3, 28, 36].

6.12 Beta-Adrenergic Receptor Antagonists

β-Adrenergic receptors have three subtypes: β_1, β_2, and β_3. Beta-1 receptors are predominantly found in two locations: the heart and the kidneys. Norepinephrine binds to the beta-1 and beta-2 receptors and activation of these receptors results in positive inotropic, dromotropic, and chronotropic effects on the heart. Activation of beta-1 receptors increases renin release from the juxtaglomerular apparatus of the kidney [47]. β-adrenergic receptor antagonists decrease blood pressure by blocking β_1 adrenergic receptors, decreasing cardiac output and inhibiting the stimulation of renin production. The cardiac-selectivity, partial agonist activity, and associated vasodilating properties of β-adrenergic receptor antagonist drugs, originated from the receptor selectivity and emphasize their pharmacodynamics properties. Some β-blockers having partial agonistic activity or intrinsic sympathomimetic activity, also having inhibitor activity both on α and β adrenergic receptors, may reduce blood pressure with a low incidence of side effects. If there isn't a problem with the electrical conduction system of the heart and cardiac functions are not impaired, β-blockers considered as safe and effective for hypertension and the incidence of OH is low [3, 28, 36, 50].

6.13 Antipsychotic Drugs

Desired pharmacological activity of antipsychotic drugs is through the blockade of dopaminergic (D_2) receptors in the central nervous system. The excess dopaminergic activity in the limbic system plays a critical role in the development of psychosis and the most of antipsychotic drugs block postsynaptic D_2 receptors especially in the mesolimbic and striatal-frontal pathways [36].Although the most of effective antipsychotic drugs block D_2 receptors, the levels of this blockade varies considerably among drugs and blockade of α adrenergic, muscarinic, H_1 histaminic, and serotonin receptors is responsible from their possible adverse reactions. Decreased baroreceptor reflex during orthostatic stress, and also decreased venous return and cardiac output may contribute to orthostatic hypotension, which is one of the clinical side effects of antipsychotic drugs [51–53]. These effects are originated from the presence of autonomic actions of these agents; manifestations of the muscarinic cholinergic receptor blockade are dry mouth, difficulty urinating and constipation, while α adrenergic receptor blockade are orthostatic hypotension.

6.14   Tricyclic Antidepressant Drugs

Antidepressants mostly focus on the monoamine hypothesis of depression suggesting that depression is related to decreased levels of serotonin, norepinephrine and dopamine as neurotransmitter in the central nervous system. Antidepressant activity of the tricyclic antidepressants (TCAs) is through the inhibition of serotonin and norepinephrine reuptake. Although the TCAs were the most important class of antidepressant agents, the use of TCAs is reserved for the patients who are unresponsive to selective serotonin reuptake inhibitors and serotonin-norepinephrine reuptake inhibitors, due to their poorer tolerability. TCAs may cause dry mouth and constipation and these adverse effects are originated to the potent anti-muscarinic actions of these drugs. However, these drugs can also act as potent antagonists of the histamine (especially H_1) receptor, causing weight gain and sedation. In addition to these, OH due to the α_1 adrenergic receptor blocker properties, is a significant adverse effect of TCAs particularly seen in older patients [28, 36, 54].

6.15   Anti-parkinsonian Drugs

Decreased dopaminergic activity in the central nervous system is the major concern for Parkinson's disease (PD) and considered as the major cause of the motor symptoms. Patients with Parkinson's disease, when compared with age-matched people in general population, generally have lower blood pressure levels. This posture related drop in blood pressure is frequently seen in PD patients, but it is generally asymptomatic [55]. Drugs used for the treatment of Parkinson's disease mainly focus on dopaminergic activity and may cause OH by interfering the autonomic or cardiovascular compensation mechanisms. OH has commonly seen and more often become symptomatic with levodopa (L-DOPA) treatment. L-DOPA is converted to dopamine and may act as a false transmitter. Also, dopamine receptor agonists may cause arterial and venous dilation by inhibiting the sympathetic activity and may aggravate OH [56–58].

6.16   Conclusion

The management of DOH is critical in elderly, concerning the higher risk of falls and its results that may adversely affect quality of life of the patients. Interdisciplinary and professional teamwork with a geriatric specialist, cardiologist and clinical pharmacologist or pharmacist should take part for the diagnosis and treatment. DOH is a frequent issue in geriatric patients and removal of the triggering factors should be the first action. Medications can be revised, decreased, changed, or stopped completely. The initial steps in the treatment of DOH are to (a) control or check the patient's inappropriate medications, (b) evaluate the patient's fluid, salt, and nutritional intake, and (c) provide patient education to prevent further problems such as falling and dizziness. Optimization of the patient's drug regime will help to ameliorate the symptoms and avoid related morbidity. Patients with diabetes mellitus, hypertension, PD, and dehydrated patients are more likely to develop OH, therefore should be closely monitored. Decent documentation of medical history is required to determine and overcome drug-induced problems. In particular, it is necessary to be very careful in treatment to prevent the development of geriatric syndromes in the elderly. If DOH attacks cannot be avoided despite discontinuation, switch or changing of the potential drugs for OH, DOH should be evaluated and treated as a primary OH.

References

1. Ricci F, De Caterina R, Fedorowski A. Orthostatic hypotension: epidemiology, prognosis, and treatment. J Am Coll Cardiol. 2015;66:848–60.
2. Mills PB, Fung CK, Travlos A, Krassioukov A. Nonpharmacologic management of orthostatic hypotension: a systematic review. Arch Phys Med Rehabil. 2015;96(2):366–75.
3. Mets TF. Drug-induced orthostatic hypotension in older patients. Drugs Aging. 1995;6(3):219–28.
4. Saedon NI, Pin Tan M, Frith J. The prevalence of orthostatic hypotension: a systematic review and meta-analysis. J Gerontol A Biol Sci Med Sci. 2020;75(1):117–22.
5. Joseph A, Wanono R, Flamant M, Vidal-Petiot E. Orthostatic hypotension: a review. Nephrol Ther. 2017;13:S55–67.
6. Méndez AS, Melgarejo JD, Mena LJ, Chávez CA, González AC, Boggia J, Terwilliger JD, Lee JH, Maestre GE. Risk factors for orthostatic hypotension: differences between elderly men and women. Am J Hypertens. 2018;31(7):797–803.
7. Low PA. Prevalence of orthostatic hypotension. Clin Auton Res. 2008;18(1):8–13.
8. Frith J, Parry SW. New horizons in orthostatic hypotension. Age Ageing. 2017;46(2):168–74.
9. Gangavati A, Hajjar I, Quach L, et al. Hypertension, orthostatic hypotension, and the risk of falls in a community-dwelling elderly population: the maintenance of balance, independent living, intellect, and zest in the elderly of Boston study. J Am Geriatr Soc. 2011;59:383–9.
10. Gupta V, Lipsitz LA. Orthostatic hypotension in the elderly: diagnosis and treatment. Am J Med. 2007;120:841–7.
11. Metzler M, Duerr S, Granata R, Krismer F, Robertson D, Wenning GK. Neurogenic orthostatic hypotension: pathophysiology, evaluation, and management. J Neurol. 2013;260(9):2212–9.
12. Gami AS, Hodge DO, Herges RM, et al. Obstructive sleep apnea, obesity, and the risk of incident atrial fibrillation. J Am Coll Cardiol. 2007;49:565–71.
13. Okin PM, Wachtell K, Kjeldsen SE, et al. Incidence of atrial fibrillation in relation to changing heart rate over time in hypertensive patients: the LIFE study. Circ Arrhythm Electrophysiol. 2008;1:337–43.
14. Nakagawa H, Scherlag BJ, Patterson E, et al. Pathophysiologic basis of autonomic ganglionated plexus ablation in patients with atrial fibrillation. Heart Rhythm. 2009;6:S26–34.
15. Fedorowski A, Burri P, Struck J, et al. Novel cardiovascular biomarkers in unexplained syncopal attacks: the SYSTEMA cohort. J Intern Med. 2013;273:359–67.

16. Berger R, Pacher R. The role of the endothelin system in myocardial infarction—new thera-peutic targets? Eur Heart J. 2003;24:294–6.
17. Kanjwal K, George A, Figueredo VM, et al. Orthostatic hypotension: definition, diagnosis and management. J Cardiovasc Med (Hagerstown). 2015;16:75–81.
18. Goldstein DS, Sharabi Y. Neurogenic orthostatic hypotension: a pathophysiological approach. Circulation. 2009;119:139–46.
19. Grubb BP, Karas B. Clinical disorders of the autonomic nervous system associated with ortho-static intolerance: an overview of classification, clinical evaluation, and management. Pacing Clin Electrophysiol. 1999;22:798–810.
20. Trahair LG, Horowitz M, Jones KL. Postprandial hypotension: a systematic review. J Am Med Dir Assoc. 2014;15:394–409.
21. Moya A, Sutton R, Ammirati F, et al. Guidelines for the diagnosis and management of syncope (version 2009). Eur Heart J. 2009;30:2631–71.
22. Poon IO, Braun U. High prevalence of orthostatic hypotension and its correlation with poten-tially causative medications among elderly veterans. J Clin Pharm Ther. 2005;30:173–8.
23. Rutan GH, Hermanson B, Bild DE, et al. Orthostatic hypotension in older adults. The cardio-vascular health study. CHS collaborative research group. Hypertension. 1992;19:508–19.
24. Bradley JG, Davis KA. Orthostatic hypotension. Am Fam Physician. 2003;68:2393–8.
25. Perez-Lloret S, Rey MV, Fabre N, et al. Factors related to orthostatic hypotension in Parkinson's disease. Parkinsonism Relat Disord. 2012;18:501–5.
26. Pathak A, Lapeyre-Mestre M, Montastruc JL, et al. Heat-related morbidity in patients with orthostatic hypotension and primary autonomic failure. Mov Disord. 2005;20:1213–9.
27. Narkiewicz K, Cooley RL, Somers VK. Alcohol potentiates orthostatic hypotension: implica-tions for alcohol-related syncope. Circulation. 2000;101:398–402.
28. Schoenberger JA. Drug-induced orthostatic hypotension. Drug Saf. 1991;6(6):402–7.
29. Freeman R, Wieling W, Axelrod FB, et al. Consensus statement on the definition of ortho-static hypotension, neurally mediated syncope and the postural tachycardia syndrome. Auton Neurosci. 2011;161:46–8.
30. Goldstein DS, Robertson D, Esler M, et al. Dysautonomias: clinical disorders of the autonomic nervous system. Ann Intern Med. 2002;137:753–63.
31. Chopra S, Baby C, Jacob JJ. Neuro-endocrine regulation of blood pressure. Indian J Endocrinol Metab. 2011;15(Suppl 4):S281–8.
32. Dampney RA, Coleman MJ, Fontes MA, et al. Central mechanisms underlying short- and long-term regulation of the cardiovascular system. Clin Exp Pharmacol Physiol. 2002;29:261–8.
33. Douglas E. Rollins, Donald K. Blumenthal. Workbook and casebook for Goodman and Gilman's the pharmacological basis of therapeutics, chapter 15: drug therapy of hypertension, edema, and disorders of sodium and water balance, © 2016, by the McGraw-Hill Companies, Inc., Printed in the United States of America.
34. Wadei HM, Textor SC. The role of the kidney in regulating arterial blood pressure. Nat Rev Nephrol. 2012;8:602–9.
35. Rhaleb NE, Yang XP, Carretero OA. The kallikrein-kinin system as a regulator of cardiovascu-lar and renal function. Compr Physiol. 2011;1:971–93.
36. Katzung BG, Trevor AJ, editors. Basic & clinical pharmacology. New York: McGraw-hill Education; 2017.
37. Perlmuter LC, Sarda G, Casavant V, Mosnaim AD. A review of the etiology, asssociated comorbidities, and treatment of orthostatic hypotension. Am J Ther. 2013;20(3):279–91.
38. Rüster C, Wolf G. Renin-angiotensin-aldosterone system and progression of renal disease. J Am Soc Nephrol. 2006;17(11):2985–91.
39. Goswami N, Blaber AP, Hinghofer-Szalkay H, Montani JP. Orthostatic intolerance in older persons: etiology and countermeasures. Front Physiol. 2017;8:803.
40. Monahan KD, Dinenno FA, Seals DR, Clevenger CM, Desouza CA, Tanaka H. Age-associated changes in cardiovagal baroreflex sensitivity are related to central arterial compliance. Am J Phys Heart Circ Phys. 2001;281(1):H284–9.

41. Juraschek SP, Daya N, Appel LJ, Miller ER, Windham BG, Pompeii L, Griswold ME, Kucharska-Newton A, Selvin E. Orthostatic hypotension in middle-age and risk of falls. Am J Hypertens. 2017;30(2):188–95.
42. Liguori I, Russo G, Coscia V, Aran L, Bulli G, Curcio F, Della-Morte D, Gargiulo G, Testa G, Cacciatore F, Bonaduce D. Orthostatic hypotension in the elderly: a marker of clinical frailty? J Am Med Dir Assoc. 2018;19(9):779–85.
43. The list of drugs with orthastatic hypotension and hypotension drug. Web application; SIDER 4.1:Side Effect Resource; 2020, January 9. http://sideeffects.embl.de/se/C0020649/
44. Finucane C, O'Connell MD, Donoghue O, et al. I mpaired orthostatic blood pressure recovery is associated with unexplained and injurious falls. J Am Geriatr Soc. 2017;65:474–82.
45. Bylund DB (2009) Norepinephrine: Adrenergic Receptors. 1231–1236.
46. Testa G, Ceccofiglio A, Mussi C, Bellelli G, Nicosia F, Bo M, Riccio D, Curcio F, Martone AM, Noro G, Landi F. Hypotensive drugs and syncope due to orthostatic hypotension in older adults with dementia (syncope and dementia study). J Am Geriatr Soc. 2018;66(8):1532–7.
47. Laurent S. Antihypertensive drugs. Pharmacol Res. 2017;124:116–25.
48. Davidson E, Fuchs J, Rotenberg Z, Weinberger I, Agmon J. Drug-related syncope. Clin Cardiol. 1989;12(10):577–80.
49. Elliott WJ, Ram CV. Calcium channel blockers. J Clin Hypertens (Greenwich). 2011;13(9):687–9.
50. Frishman WH. Beta-adrenergic receptor blockers. Adverse effects and drug interactions. Hypertension. 1988;11(3):21–9.
51. White WB. Hypotension with postural syncope secondary to the combination of chlorpromazine and captopril. Arch Intern Med. 1986;146(9):1833–4.
52. Takata Y, Kurihara J, Suzuki S, Okubo Y, Kato H. A rabbit model for evaluation of chlorpromazine-induced orthostatic Shypotension. Biol Pharm Bull. 1999;22(5):457–62.
53. Nourian Z, Mow T, Muftic D, Burek S, Pedersen ML, Matz J, Mulvany MJ. Orthostatic hypotensive effect of antipsychotic drugs in Wistar rats by in vivo and in vitro studies of α 1-adrenoceptor function. Psychopharmacology. 2008;199(1):15.
54. Briggs R, Carey D, McNicholas T, Claffey P, Nolan H, Kennelly SP, Kenny RA. The association between antidepressant use and orthostatic hypotension in older people: a matched cohort study. J Am Soc Hypertens. 2018;12(8):597–604.
55. Mcdowell FH, Lee JE. Levodopa, Parkinson's disease, and hypotension. Ann Intern Med. 1970;72(5):751–2.
56. Kujawa K, Leurgans S, Raman R, Blasucci L, Goetz CG. Acute orthostatic hypotension when starting dopamine agonists in Parkinson's disease. Arch Neurol. 2000;57(10):1461–3.
57. Mehagnoul-Schipper DJ, Boerman RH, Hoefnagels WH, Jansen RW. Effect of levodopa on orthostatic and postprandial hypotension in elderly parkinsonian patients. J Gerontol Ser A Biol Med Sci. 2001;56(12):M749–55.
58. Piha SJ, Rinne JO, Rinne UK, Seppänen A. Autonomic dysfunction in recent onset and advanced Parkinson's disease. Clin Neurol Neurosurg. 1988;90(3):221–6.

Comorbidities and Geriatric Syndromes Related to Orthostatic Hypotension

Lee Smith and Pinar Soysal

7.1 Frailty and Orthostatic Hypotension

Frailty is characterized by the reduction of a physiological reserve and the ability to resist physical or psychological stresses [1–4]. There is a small but growing body of literature that shows frailty is associated with OH. In a study of 496 Turkish patients, who were admitted to a geriatric clinic, using a cross-sectional observational study design, individuals classified as frail were more likely to have OH compared to those categorized as frail and robust [5]. In another study of 116 participants residing in a long-term care facility and 65 years and over it was found that in frail individuals the prevalence of initial OH, recovery OH, consensus OH and delayed OH was 15, 12, 56 and 49%, respectively. In non-frail individuals, the prevalence of initial OH, recovery OH, consensus OH and delayed OH was 4, 0, 32 and 48% [6]. In a cross-sectional study of 693 older patients admitted to a geriatric evaluation and management unit multivariate logistic regression showed a significant association between OH and frailty, but the association attenuated after adjustment for physical function. Nevertheless, associations between OH and frailty remained significant among vulnerable subgroups such as women, subjects having weakness, slowness, poor cognitive function, polypharmacy or any Instrumental Activities of Daily Living limitation [7]. Several other studies have found similar findings [8–10].

There are several plausible pathways that may explain the observed association between OH and frailty. First, frailty is associated with impaired autonomic cardiovascular control and damage to the autonomic nervous system may result in OH [1,

L. Smith
The Cambridge Centre for Sport and Exercise Sciences, Anglia Ruskin University, Cambridge, UK
e-mail: lee.smith@aru.ac.uk

P. Soysal (✉)
Department of Geriatric Medicine, Faculty of Medicine, Bezmialem Vakif University, Istanbul, Turkey

© Springer Nature Switzerland AG 2021
A. T. Isik, P. Soysal (eds.), *Orthostatic Hypotension in Older Adults*,
https://doi.org/10.1007/978-3-030-62493-4_7

11, 12]. Moreover, decreased baroreceptor sensitivity may be a contributing factor in older adults and baroreceptor responsiveness is likely to be deteriorated earlier in frail people [13]. Second, OH has been associated with poor peripheral motor nerve function in old age [14]. Slower gait speed as a part of frailty may be linked to impaired orthostatic response. Decreased calf blood flow may impair the upright ejective ability of the skeletal muscle to pump and further contributes to the overall reduced blood flow and orthostatic intolerance in these patients [15]. Moreover, a decrease in muscle mass resulting in frailty may lead to OH by increasing venous pooling. Third, the anti-muscarinic effect of atropinic drugs can cause significant OH [16, 17]. Consequently, the anti-muscarinic effect can be a shared mechanism for frailty and OH. Fourth, inflammation is a common mechanism in frailty. Frailty and pre-frailty are associated with higher inflammatory parameters [18]. In the literature, OH may be independently associated with systemic inflammation in non-diabetic adults [19]. As a result, inflammation can be a shared mechanism to account for the relationship between frailty and OH.

Frailty status might be a risk factor for OH, and both OH and frailty may interplay and affect each other. Since frailty can exacerbate age-related physiological changes and is usually associated with other comorbidities and drugs, OH may occur in the early period by disrupting the compensatory responses to orthostatic changes. Therefore, changes in orthostatic blood pressure in the first minute may have higher clinical significance for frail older adults.

7.2   Dementia and Orthostatic Hypotension

Dementia may be defined as a set of symptoms that may include memory loss and difficulties with thinking, problem-solving or language [20]. Dementia occurs when the brain is damaged by diseases such as Alzheimer's disease (AD) [21]. Moreover, mild cognitive impairment is considered the precursor of dementia. There is a growing body of literature to suggest that OH is associated with dementia. A 12-year follow-up study found that there was at least a 25% increase in risk between OH presence of 7425 participants aged 65 and over and dementia during follow-up [22]. In the Rotterdam study among 6204 participants (mean ± standard deviation [SD] age 68.5 ± 8.6 years) with a median follow-up of 15.3 years it was found that OH was associated with an increased risk of dementia, which was similar for AD and vascular dementia [23]. In another study of 495 older adults aged 76 ± 8 years of age, after adjusting for age, education level, systolic BP, diastolic BP, weight, and antihypertensive drugs, subjects with OH had a worse cognitive function than those without OH. Moreover, the study found that OH was present in 22% of participants with vascular dementia, 15% in those with AD, 12% in those with mild cognitive impairment and 4% in those without cognitive impairment or dementia [24]. Several other studies have also demonstrated that OH is associated with dementia and mild cognitive impairment [25, 26].

There are several plausible pathways that may explain the relationship between OH and risk of mild cognitive impairment and dementia. First, the same cerebral areas involved in the neurodegenerative process leading to dementia syndromes are devoted to the autonomic control of the cardiovascular system, thus neurodegeneration can be the cause of both cognitive impairment and OH [27]. Second, OH may result in cerebral hypoperfusion which plays a role in the development of cognitive impairment [25]. Autonomic nervous system function is responsible for maintaining continuous cerebral perfusion, together with local vasoreactivity, which has previously been associated with the risk of dementia in the general population. Brief episodes of hypoperfusion elicited by sudden blood pressure drops may lead to hypoxia, with detrimental effects on brain tissue via, for instance, neuroinflammation and oxidative stress [23]. Finally, OH serves as a marker of other detrimental consequences of autonomic dysfunction, such as blood pressure variability, response to Valsalva manoeuvre, cardiovascular reflex and heart rate variability, and 30/15 ratio. Several of these measures may be linked to dementia via hypoperfusion, but other pathways could be involved also. For example, decreased compliance of the arterial wall with hypertension may contribute to OH by reducing baroreceptor sensitivity. Arterial stiffness and OH are both associated with increased burden of cerebral white matter lesions and vascular disease including stroke, which are risk factors for dementia [23].

Dementia with Lewy Bodies (DLB) is the second most common dementia, after Alzheimer's disease (AD), with a clinical prevalence of 15–42% of all dementia cases [28] and previous studies have demonstrated that prevalence of OH has been reported in 42–69% of patients with DLB [29]. Therefore, due to the high prevalence, OH is considered one of the supporting clinical features of the disease, along with other symptoms of autonomic dysfunction, such as constipation and urinary incontinence [30]. Actually, autonomic dysfunctions are well known as part of all alpha-synucleinopathies, including Multiple System Atrophy (MSA), DLB, and Parkinson's Disease (PD), due to the presence of Lewy bodies in brain regions such as Locus coeruleus [25]. However, despite the fact that OH, as a sign of autonomic dysfunction, might also help in differential diagnosis among dementia subtypes, it should be kept in mind that autonomic dysfunction is common in all forms of dementia [25, 31], and reported prevalence of OH is between 33% and 42% in patients with AD whereas it is between 13% and 14% in healthy controls [29, 32]. In AD, it has been reported that both generalized deficit in cholinergic function and the involvement of the subcortical structures, implicated in autonomic nervous system regulation, may lead to autonomic dysfunction in the course of the disease. Indeed, a study by Isik et al. showed that the frequency of OH in patients with AD is similar to those with DLB [33].

OH causes several negative health consequences including cardiovascular events, falls, fractures, progression of dementia, and mortality in older adults [34]. Moreover, it can be considered as a marker or risk factor of clinical frailty. Therefore, clinicians should be aware of OH and its associated consequences in the treatment of dementia patients.

7.3   Depression and Orthostatic Hypotension

Depression (major depressive disorder or clinical depression) is a common but serious mood disorder. It causes severe symptoms that affect how one feels, thinks, and handles daily activities, such as sleeping and eating [35]. There is a growing body of literature to suggest that there is a relationship between depression and OH. Indeed, OH has been shown to be highly prevalent (51.3%) in those with late-life depression [36]. Another study found similar findings [37]. However, it should be noted that in this study the prevalence of OH in those with depression varied depending on the measure used to determine OH. One study aimed to investigate the longitudinal association between baseline symptomatic OH (sOH) and incident depression in a sample of >3000 older people (mean age 62 years) without baseline depression. The study found that sOH predicts incident depression in a population-representative sample of older people and may, therefore, represent a potentially modifiable risk factor for late-life depression [38]. Another study revealed a significantly greater systolic and diastolic blood pressure drop in antidepressant users than nonusers at 30 s after standing. The prevalence of OH among antidepressant users was 31% (63/206), compared with 17% in nonusers [39]. Other studies have also found a relationship between depression and OH [40, 41].

Several mechanisms may explain the relationship between OH and depression. Given the strong vascular basis of late life depression, as well as the structural brain changes associated with this, one would expect to find a close relationship with blood pressure control [41]. Indeed, patients with late-life depression have been shown to have higher rates of cerebrovascular disease, reflected by cerebral white matter disease, than patients with earlier onset depression [42]. Hypotension can be an end-point for several diverse disease processes in the older person, including congestive heart failure and lung disease. Rates of depression are also significantly higher in older people with more profound chronic medical illness. Therefore, it may be that both depression and OH are markers of poor physical health, which mediates the relationship between the two [41].

7.4   Sarcopenia and Orthostatic Hypotension

Sarcopenia, one of the geriatric syndromes, has attracted attention over the last three decades [43]. Although revised criteria for sarcopenia were published in 2019, the number of studies using these criteria is small. In a recent study, it was found that 40% of the patients had no sarcopenia, whereas 11% had severe sarcopenia according to new criteria [44]. The high prevalence of sarcopenia is remarkable in older adults because sarcopenia is known not only as a simple muscle disease but also to affect many organ systems, particularly the respiratory and cardiovascular system.

Not surprisingly, sarcopenia and the severity of is associated with the development of OH, which can be explained by several mechanisms: First, sarcopenia can lead to a reduction in effective venous return, since venous pumps in the leg muscles pump blood from the lower extremity to the heart, which is important in maintaining cardiac filling pressure [45]. To date there is no study investigating the relationship between sarcopenia and OH. However, some studies indirectly support this. For example, Suzuki et al., using a sample of young adults, reported that there was a decrease in venous return and cardiac output following 20-day bed rest, due to the decrease in muscle mass and muscle strength, and that patients had deterioration in orthostatic tolerance capacity [46]. In another study, it was found that calf circumference, which has a negative close correlation with appendicular skeletal muscle mass, could be used for OH screening in older adults [47]. Moreover, isometric contraction of the muscles under the waist, which plays a role in maintaining blood pressure when one stands-up by increasing venous return, is recommended for the prevention of OH [48]. This maneuver, which is well known for its effect on OH management, may indicate the importance of muscle mass and sarcopenia in the development of OH. Besides, in a study including 37 patients, sarcopenia was diagnosed by Skeletal Muscle Index (SMI); lower systolic blood pressure was more common in those with, rather than those without, sarcopenia. However, there was no correlation with OH, which may be owing to the low sample size of the study [49]. The results of these studies reporting that there may be a close relationship between sarcopenia and OH, suggest that it is a consequence in a reduction of skeletal muscle mass rather than muscle strength. Moreover, in older adults, OH may play a role in the reduction of muscle mass and sarcopenia by causing falls, balance and gait problems, and possibly making patients less mobile [34]. However, further studies are needed to identify if longitudinal associations exist between sarcopenia and OH.

7.5   Malnutrition and Orthostatic Hypotension

Malnutrition, which is frequently seen in older adults, causes negative serious outcomes. Prevalence of malnutrition is 5–10% in community-dwelling older adults, 30–61% in hospitalized older patients and 12–85% in nursing homes [50]. Malnutrition, increases the risk of infection, sarcopenia, frailty, pressure injury, falls, fracture and mortality, causing a delay in immune response and wound healing [51]. Despite all these negative effects, malnutrition, a disorder that can often be overlooked, remains a significant and frequent public health problem [52]. Therefore, regular nutritional status screening should be recommended in older adults [52, 53]. However, the relationship between OH and malnutrition and/or the risk of malnutrition is unknown.

A recent study by Kocyigit et al. retrospectively evaluated 862 older patients and found that both malnutrition and malnutrition-risk might be related to systolic OH in older adults [50]. It was also found that malnutrition-risk may be predictive for OH. The results of this study may be explained through several hypotheses. First, the mechanism that may explain the relationship between malnutrition and systolic OH may be autonomic dysfunction [54]. According to a meta-analysis describing the causes of aging, anorexia was reported to be involved in the etiopathogenesis of autonomic dysfunction [54]. Autonomic neuropathy also may play a role in the aetiology of OH [55], as systolic OH may be associated with sympathetic failure

[56]. Second, it is known that systolic OH is caused by impaired peripheral vaso-constriction [56]. Sarcopenia is a geriatric syndrome leading to loss of muscle mass. A working groups' consensus proposed to define sarcopenia as a syndrome characterized by age-related loss of muscle mass and loss of muscle function, including muscle mass and strength and/or physical performance [57]. In one study, parameters of malnutrition were shown to be related with diagnostic measures of sarcopenia in geriatric outpatients and the association between parameters of malnutrition and diagnostic measures of sarcopenia was significant for both relative and absolute muscle mass [58]. Influence of nutrition-related reduction in muscle mass and muscle tone in vascular muscle mass may also signify the association.

Interestingly, micronutrient deficiency can also lead to OH, and especially vitamin D deficiency and vitamin B12 deficiency. However, the results of the studies on this subject are not compatible. In one study involving 546 elderly patients, Soysal et al. found that the frequency of OH in those with vitamin D deficiency was significantly higher than those without vitamin D deficiency [59]. Vitamin D deficiency is thought to cause a decrease in baroreceptor sensitivity and increase arterial stiffness, disrupting the regulation of the renin angiotensin aldosterone system and creating a trend for OH development [59]. However, in another study, this relationship could not be shown, while in another, the OH–Vitamin D deficiency relationship was found only in oldest women [60]. Finally, 12-month high-dose vitamin D replacement was found to be ineffective in treating OH [59]. In vitamin B12 deficiency, as with diabetic neuropathy, OH may be observed due to myelination defect of autonomic nervous system involvement and postganglionic nerve fibres. Moreover, OH improvement has been shown after vitamin B12 replacement [61]. Taken together these findings support that nutritional factors can cause OH, thus patients with OH should be screened for malnutrition risk and malnutrition, and serum levels of micronutrients should be kept to an optimum level.

7.6   Falls/Fear of Falling and Orthostatic Hypotension

Fear of falling (FoF) and falling per se are two important health problems for older adults. Equivalent to the aetiology of OH, fall risk is a complex and multifactorial phenomenon and OH is one of the many risk factors to contribute to an increased fall rate and FoF in older adults [62].

Both OH and FoF/falls have many common adverse outcomes such as cognitive impairment, functional impairments, depression, and poor quality of life [62]. However, the number of studies investigating the relationship between these two health outcomes is limited, and the direction of the association is not known, that is whether FoF leads to OH or whether OH leads to FoF. Nevertheless, some possible mechanisms can explain this relationship. Depending on OH, problems with gait and balance in older adults can lead to decreased functionality, thus resulting in physical inactivity and consequently may contribute to the development of falls and FoF. OH causes sudden reduction in brain perfusion and oxygenation within a few minutes of postural change; this may result in symptoms such as dizziness, postural lightheadedness, vertigo, and blurred vision in those with OH [63]. Moreover, OH causes impaired muscle microcirculation and pain in the neck, hip and calf muscles [64].Importantly, chronic brain pathology, such as brain atrophy, microbleeds, and white matter brain lesions are more common in those with OH; which might influence the perception of verticality, resulting in positive dizziness. Taken together, these potential mechanisms may explain how OH can cause falls and FoF.

FOF/falls has been identified as an independent risk factor for reduced quality of life, activity restriction, loss of independence, and a leading cause of injury, morbidity, and mortality [65]. As a result, those who have FoF/recurrent falls, begin to limit their daily activities in order not to fall again, and consequently, there may be a decrease in muscle strength and balance abilities. The reduced muscle mass and muscle strength can lead to a reduction in effective venous return, since venous pumps in the leg muscles pump blood from the lower extremity to the heart, which is important in maintaining cardiac filling pressure [66]. For example, Suzuki et al., in young subjects, reported that there was a decrease in venous return and cardiac output following 20-day bed rest, due to the decrease in muscle mass and muscle strength, and that patients had deterioration in orthostatic tolerance capacity [46]. Accordingly, FoF and falls can be a risk factor for OH in older adults.

7.7 Orthostatic Hypotension and Comorbidities

Simply put a comorbidity is the presence of one or more additional conditions co-occurring with a primary condition. There is a growing body of literature to suggest the OH is associated with a higher risk of comorbidity.

Cardiovascular disease (CVD) is the name for the group of disorders of heart and blood vessels, and includes hypertension, coronary heart disease, cerebrovascular disease, peripheral vascular disease, heart failure, rheumatic heart disease, congenital heart disease, and cardiomyopathies. A relatively large body of literature suggests that OH is associated with CVD. For example, in a systematic review of 28 prospective studies nine prospective studies found an association between OH and cardiovascular events including coronary disease, heart failure, and arrhythmias [67]. However, insufficient data were available to enable a precise assessment of the association of OH with strokes [67]. In a more recent review including 15 prospective cohort studies, subjects with OH had a high risk of heart failure and atrial fibrillation. Moreover, significant associations were found between OH and risks of developing coronary heart disease and myocardial infarction [67].

Moreover, in a recent study examining the long-term association between OH and risk of stroke in a sample of 11,709 participants, it was found that over ≈25 years, 842 had an ischemic stroke. Compared to persons without OH at baseline, those with OH had a higher risk of ischemic stroke. The study concludes that OH assessed in midlife was independently associated with incident ischemic stroke [68]. It should be noted that cardiovascular and coronary events have been shown to be more closely linked with diastolic OH than systolic. Indeed, coronary circulation may be reduced in people with diastolic OH. The increased vascular inflammatory process, peripheral artery disease, and higher dyslipidaemia, found in patients with OH compared to those without OH, likely contributes to higher risk of cardiovascular/coronary disease/events [67]. Moreover, the presence of OH has been shown to be associated with left ventricular myocardial hypertrophy and increased intima-media thickness [69].

7.8   Orthostatic Hypotension and Mortality

Interestingly, OH has been shown to be associated with mortality. A meta-analysis of seven prospective studies found that OH was associated with a significant increased risk for overall mortality [67]. Another study concluded that more pronounced orthostatic blood pressure drop predicted higher mortality, and increased mortality in OH was associated with both systolic and diastolic disruption [70]. Perhaps the key driver between OH and mortality is cerebral hypoperfusion. A decrease in blood pressure and/or cardiac output results in cerebral hypoperfusion and cerebral hypoperfusion can cause a range of brain injuries [70].

OH represents a condition of impaired hemodynamic homeostasis, where compensatory neuroendocrine mechanisms are intermittently activated. These mechanisms may trigger the activation of other biologic effectors, e.g., platelets or the coagulation cascade, potentially promoting the occurrence of cardio- or cerebrovascular events that can contribute to a higher mortality risk [19, 69]. Moreover, wide swings in blood pressure and supine hypertension associated with OH may provoke intermittent ischemic bouts and increased afterload, leading to permanent end-organ damage such as left ventricular hypertrophy and decreased renal function [63]. Baroreflex dysfunction, a marker of autonomic nervous system imbalance implicated in the pathogenesis of OH is characterized by enhanced sympathetic activity and withdrawal of parasympathetic control and has long been recognized as an important mediator of increased cardiovascular morbidity and mortality.

References

1. Joseph A, Wanono R, Flamant M, Vidal-Petiot E. Orthostatic hypotension: a review. Nephrol Ther. 2017;13(Suppl 1):S55–67.
2. Valderas JM, Starfield B, Sibbald B, Salisbury C, Roland M. Defining comorbidity: implications for understanding health and health services. Ann Fam Med. 2009;7(4):357–63.
3. Inouye SK, Studenski S, Tinetti ME, Kuchel GA. Geriatric syndromes: clinical, research, and policy implications of a core geriatric concept. J Am Geriatr Soc. 2007;55(5):780–91.
4. Bergman H, Ferrucci L, Guralnik J, Hogan DB, Hummel S, Karunananthan S, et al. Frailty: an emerging research and clinical paradigm--issues and controversies. J Gerontol A Biol Sci Med Sci. 2007;62(7):731–7.
5. Kocyigit SE, Soysal P, Bulut EA, Aydin AE, Dokuzlar O, Isik AT. What is the relationship between frailty and orthostatic hypotension in older adults? J Geriatr Cardiol. 2019;16(3):272–9.
6. Shaw BH, Borrel D, Sabbaghan K, Kum C, Yang Y, Robinovitch SN, et al. Relationships between orthostatic hypotension, frailty, falling and mortality in elderly care home residents. BMC Geriatr. 2019;19(1):80.

7. Chen L, Xu Y, Chen X-J, Lee W-J, Chen L-K. Association between orthostatic hypotension and frailty in hospitalized older patients: a geriatric syndrome more than a cardiovascular condition. J Nutr Health Aging. 2019;23:318–22.
8. Ooi WL, Barrett S, Hossain M, Kelley-Gagnon M, Lipsitz LA. Patterns of orthostatic blood pressure change and their clinical correlates in a frail, elderly population. JAMA. 1997;277(16):1299–304.
9. Liguori I, Russo G, Coscia V, Aran L, Bulli G, Curcio F, et al. Orthostatic hypotension in the elderly: a marker of clinical frailty? J Am Med Dir Assoc. 2018;19(9):779–85.
10. Indani H, Bansal R, Chatterjee P, Chakrawarty A, Dwivedi S, Dey AB. Orthostatic hypotension and its relationship with frailty. Innov Aging. 2017;1:1130.
11. Varadhan R, Chaves PHM, Lipsitz LA, Stein PK, Tian J, Windham BG, et al. Frailty and impaired cardiac autonomic control: new insights from principal components aggregation of traditional heart rate variability indices. J Gerontol A Biol Sci Med Sci. 2009;64(6):682–7.
12. Katayama PL, Dias DPM, Silva LEV, Virtuoso-Junior JS, Marocolo M. Cardiac autonomic modulation in non-frail, pre-frail and frail elderly women: a pilot study. Aging Clin Exp Res. 2015;27(5):621–9.
13. Kithas PA, Supiano MA. Hypertension in the geriatric population: a patient-centered approach. Med Clin North Am. 2015;99(2):379–89.
14. O'Connell MD, Savva GM, Finucane C, Romero-Ortuno R, Fan CW, Kenny RA. Impairments in hemodynamic responses to Orthostasis associated with frailty: results from the Irish longitudinal study on Ageing (TILDA). J Am Geriatr Soc. 2018;66(8):1475–83.
15. Stewart JM, Medow MS, Montgomery LD, McLeod K. Decreased skeletal muscle pump activity in patients with postural tachycardia syndrome and low peripheral blood flow. Am J Physiol Heart Circ Physiol. 2004;286(3):H1216–22.
16. Li H, Kem DC, Reim S, Khan M, Vanderlinde-Wood M, Zillner C, et al. Agonistic auto-antibodies as vasodilators in orthostatic hypotension: a new mechanism. Hypertension. 2012;59(2):402–8.
17. Moulis F, Moulis G, Balardy L, Gerard S, Montastruc F, Sourdet S, et al. Exposure to atropinic drugs and frailty status. J Am Med Dir Assoc. 2015;16(3):253–7.
18. Soysal P, Stubbs B, Lucato P, Luchini C, Solmi M, Peluso R, et al. Inflammation and frailty in the elderly: a systematic review and meta-analysis. Ageing Res Rev. 2016;31:1–8.
19. Fedorowski A, Ostling G, Persson M, Struck J, Engstrom G, Nilsson PM, et al. Orthostatic blood pressure response, carotid intima-media thickness, and plasma fibrinogen in older non-diabetic adults. J Hypertens. 2012;30(3):522–9.
20. Soysal P, Usarel C, Ispirli G, Isik AT. Attended with and head-turning sign can be clinical markers of cognitive impairment in older adults. Int Psychogeriatr. 2017;29(11):1569.
21. Isik AT. Late onset Alzheimer's disease in older people. Clin Interv Aging. 2010;5:307–11.
22. Cremer A, Soumare A, Berr C, Dartigues J-F, Gabelle A, Gosse P, et al. Orthostatic hypotension and risk of incident dementia: results from a 12-year follow-up of the Three-City study cohort. Hypertension. 2017;70(1):44–9.
23. Wolters FJ, Mattace-Raso FUS, Koudstaal PJ, Hofman A, Ikram MA. Orthostatic hypotension and the long-term risk of dementia: a population-based study. PLoS Med. 2016;13(10):e1002143.
24. Mehrabian S, Duron E, Labouree F, Rollot F, Bune A, Traykov L, et al. Relationship between orthostatic hypotension and cognitive impairment in the elderly. J Neurol Sci. 2010;299(1–2):45–8.
25. Sambati L, Calandra-Buonaura G, Poda R, Guaraldi P, Cortelli P. Orthostatic hypotension and cognitive impairment: a dangerous association? Neurol Sci. 2014;35(6):951–7.
26. Perlmuter LC, Sarda G, Casavant V, O'Hara K, Hindes M, Knott PT, et al. A review of orthostatic blood pressure regulation and its association with mood and cognition. Clin Auton Res. 2012;22(2):99–107.
27. Del Pino R, Murueta-Goyena A, Acera M, Carmona-Abellan M, Tijero B, Lucas-Jimenez O, et al. Autonomic dysfunction is associated with neuropsychological impairment in Lewy body disease. J Neurol. 2020;267(7):1941–51.

28. Mueller C, Soysal P, Rongve A, Isik AT, Thompson T, Maggi S, et al. Survival time and differences between dementia with Lewy bodies and Alzheimer's disease following diagnosis: a meta-analysis of longitudinal studies. Ageing Res Rev. 2019;50:72–80.
29. Andersson M, Hansson O, Minthon L, Ballard CG, Londos E. The period of hypotension following orthostatic challenge is prolonged in dementia with Lewy bodies. Int J Geriatr Psychiatry. 2008;23(2):192–8.
30. McKeith IG, Boeve BF, DIckson DW, Halliday G, Taylor JP, Weintraub D, et al. Diagnosis and management of dementia with Lewy bodies: fourth consensus report of the DLB consortium. Neurology. 2017;89(1):88–100.
31. O'Callaghan S, Kenny RA. Neurocardiovascular instability and cognition. Yale J Biol Med. 2016;89(1):59–71.
32. Sonnesyn H, Nilsen DW, Rongve A, Nore S, Ballard C, Tysnes OB, et al. High prevalence of orthostatic hypotension in mild dementia. Dement Geriatr Cogn Disord. 2009;28(4):307–13.
33. Isik AT, Kocyigit SE, Smith L, Aydin AE, Soysal P. A comparison of the prevalence of orthostatic hypotension between older patients with Alzheimer's disease, Lewy body dementia, and without dementia. Exp Gerontol. 2019;124:110628.
34. Soysal P, Veronese N, Smith L, Torbahn G, Jackson SE, Yang L, et al. Orthostatic hypotension and health outcomes: an umbrella review of observational studies. Eur Geriatric Med. 2019;10:863–870.
35. Soysal P, Veronese N, Thompson T, Kahl KG, Fernandes BS, Prina AM, et al. Relationship between depression and frailty in older adults: a systematic review and meta-analysis. Ageing Res Rev. 2017;36:78–87.
36. Vasudev A, O'Brien JT, Tan MP, Parry SW, Thomas AJ. A study of orthostatic hypotension, heart rate variability and baroreflex sensitivity in late-life depression. J Affect Disord. 2011;131(1–3):374–8.
37. Shanbhag A, Awai H, Rej S, Thomas AJ, Puka K, Vasudev A. Orthostatic hypotension in patients with late-life depression: prevalence and validation of a new screening tool. Int J Geriatr Psychiatry. 2018;33(10):1397–402.
38. Briggs R, Carey D, Kennelly SP, Kenny RA. Longitudinal association between orthostatic hypotension at 30 seconds post-standing and late-life depression. Hypertension. 2018;71(5):946–54.
39. Briggs R, Carey D, McNicholas T, Claffey P, Nolan H, Kennelly SP, et al. The association between antidepressant use and orthostatic hypotension in older people: a matched cohort study. J Am Soc Hypertens. 2018;12(8):597–604.e1.
40. Richardson J, Kerr SRJ, Shaw F, Kenny RA, O'Brien JT, Thomas AJ. A study of orthostatic hypotension in late-life depression. Am J Geriatr Psychiatry. 2009;17(11):996–9.
41. Briggs R, Kenny RA, Kennelly SP. Systematic review: the association between late life depression and hypotension. J Am Med Dir Assoc. 2016;17(12):1076–88.
42. Krishnan KR, McDonald WM. Arteriosclerotic depression. Med Hypotheses. 1995;44(2):111–5.
43. Cruz-Jentoft AJ, Bahat G, Bauer J, Boirie Y, Bruyere O, Cederholm T, et al. Sarcopenia: revised European consensus on definition and diagnosis. Age Ageing. 2019;48(1):16–31.
44. Soysal, P. Kocyigit SE, Ozge Dokuzlar, Esra Ates Bulut, Lee Smith Ahmet Turan Isik. Relationship between sarcopenia and orthostatic hypotension in older adults. Age Ageing. 2020; Inpress.
45. Rowell LB. Human cardiovascular control. 1st ed. Oxford: Oxford University Press; 1993.
46. Suzuki Y, Murakami T, Kawakubo K, Haruna Y, Takenaka K, Goto S, et al. Regional changes in muscle mass and strength following 20 days of bed rest, and the effects on orthostatic tolerance capacity in young subjects. J Gravit Physiol. 1994;1(1):P57–8.
47. Kobayashi K, Yamada S. Development of a simple index, calf mass index, for screening for orthostatic hypotension in community-dwelling elderly. Arch Gerontol Geriatr. 2012;54(2):293–7.
48. Figueroa JJ, Basford JR, Low PA. Preventing and treating orthostatic hypotension: as easy as a, B, C. Cleve Clin J Med. 2010;77(5):298–306.

49. Shanahan E, Sheehy T, Costelloe A, Peters C, Lyons D, O'Connor M. 221 relationship between skeletal muscle mass and orthostatic hypotension. Age Ageing. 2016;45(suppl_2):ii13–56. https://doi.org/10.1093/ageing/afw159.199.
50. Kocyigit SE, Soysal P, Ates Bulut E, Isik AT. Malnutrition and malnutrition risk can be associated with systolic orthostatic hypotension in older adults. J Nutr Health Aging. 2018;22(8):928–33.
51. Soderstrom L, Rosenblad A, Thors Adolfsson E, Bergkvist L. Malnutrition is associated with increased mortality in older adults regardless of the cause of death. Br J Nutr. 2017;117(4):532–40.
52. Visvanathan R, Newbury JW, Chapman I. Malnutrition in older people--screening and management strategies. Aust Fam Physician. 2004;33(10):799–805.
53. Kalan U, Arik F, Isik AT, Soysal P. Nutritional profiles of older adults according the mini-nutritional assessment. Aging Clin Exp Res. 2020;32(4):673–80.
54. Roy M, Gaudreau P, Payette H. A scoping review of anorexia of aging correlates and their relevance to population health interventions. Appetite. 2016;105:688–99.
55. Frith J, Parry SW. New horizons in orthostatic hypotension. Age Ageing. 2017;46(2):168–74.
56. Luukinen H, Koski K, Laippala P, Kivela SL. Prognosis of diastolic and systolic orthostatic hypotension in older persons. Arch Intern Med. 1999;159(3):273–80.
57. Cruz-Jentoft AJ, Baeyens JP, Bauer JM, Boirie Y, Cederholm T, Landi F, et al. Sarcopenia: european consensus on definition and diagnosis: report of the european working group on sarcopenia in older people. Age Ageing. 2010;39(4):412–23. http://www.ncbi.nlm.nih.gov/pubmed/20392703%5Cn, http://www.pubmedcentral.nih.gov/articlerender.fcgi?artid=PMC2886201
58. Reijnierse EM, Trappenburg MC, Leter MJ, Blauw GJ, de van der Schueren MAE, CGM M, et al. The association between parameters of malnutrition and diagnostic measures of sarcopenia in geriatric outpatients. PLoS One. 2015;10(8):e0135933.
59. Soysal P, Yay A, Isik AT. Does vitamin D deficiency increase orthostatic hypotension risk in the elderly patients? Arch Gerontol Geriatr. 2014;59(1):74–7.
60. Annweiler C, Schott A-M, Rolland Y, Beauchet O. Vitamin D deficiency is associated with orthostatic hypotension in oldest-old women. J Intern Med. 2014;276(3):285–95.
61. Moore A, Ryan J, Watts M, Pillay I, Clinch D, Lyons D. Orthostatic tolerance in older patients with vitamin B12 deficiency before and after vitamin B12 replacement. Clin Auton Res. 2004;14(2):67–71.
62. Makino K, Makizako H, Doi T, Tsutsumimoto K, Hotta R, Nakakubo S, et al. Impact of fear of falling and fall history on disability incidence among older adults: prospective cohort study. Int J Geriatr Psychiatry. 2018;33(4):658–62.
63. Low PA, Opfer-Gehrking TL, McPhee BR, Fealey RD, Benarroch EE, Willner CL, et al. Prospective evaluation of clinical characteristics of orthostatic hypotension. Mayo Clin Proc. 1995;70(7):617–22.
64. Bleasdale-Barr KM, Mathias CJ. Neck and other muscle pains in autonomic failure: their association with orthostatic hypotension. J R Soc Med. 1998;91(7):355–9.
65. Young WR, Mark Williams A. How fear of falling can increase fall-risk in older adults: applying psychological theory to practical observations. Gait Posture. 2015;41(1):7–12.
66. Rowel LB. Human cardiovascular control. 1th ed. Oxford: Oxford University Press; 1993.
67. Angelousi A, Girerd N, Benetos A, Frimat L, Gautier S, Weryha G, et al. Association between orthostatic hypotension and cardiovascular risk, cerebrovascular risk, cognitive decline and falls as well as overall mortality: a systematic review and meta-analysis. J Hypertens. 2014;32(8):1562–71; discussion 1571
68. Rawlings AM, Juraschek SP, Heiss G, Hughes T, Meyer ML, Selvin E, et al. Association of orthostatic hypotension with incident dementia, stroke, and cognitive decline. Neurology. 2018;91(8):e759–68.

69. Fan X-H, Wang Y, Sun K, Zhang W, Wang H, Wu H, et al. Disorders of orthostatic blood pressure response are associated with cardiovascular disease and target organ damage in hypertensive patients. Am J Hypertens. 2010;23(8):829–37.
70. Fedorowski A, Stavenow L, Hedblad B, Berglund G, Nilsson PM, Melander O. Orthostatic hypotension predicts all-cause mortality and coronary events in middle-aged individuals (the Malmo preventive project). Eur Heart J. 2010;31(1):85–91.

Orthostatic Hypotension in Neurodegenerative Diseases

Neziha Erken and Ahmet Turan Isik

Orthostatic hypotension (OH) is a geriatric syndrome that affects daily life activities and impairs quality of life. As soon as the person stands up, it is the clinical reflection of hemostatic insufficiency that develops as a result of not being able to pump enough blood from peripheral tissue to the center due to the disruption of coordination of the cardiovascular structures, musculoskeletal system, endocrine and nervous system [1]. After standing up with the effect of gravity, approximately 500–1000 mL of blood are deposited in the lower extremitiesand splanchnic area; therefore, cardiac output and blood pressure (BP) decrease. Baroreceptors in the carotid sinus and aortic arch are stimulated. Through compensatory reflex, sympathetic tone increases, while parasympathetic tone decreases. With vascular resistance in the peripheral, 50% of the blood is sent back to the heart in 2 or 3 s, by which blood pressure drop is prevented. If the compensatory reflex system is disrupted, OH appears [2, 3].

OH, also a common condition in the course of various neurodegenerative diseases, is defined as neurogenic OH (nOH) when caused by neurodegenerative processes. nOH is considered as one of the clinical outcomes of autonomic dysfunction caused by a neurodegenerative process [2]. As seen in Fig. 8.1, nOH may be due to peripheral causes or it may develop as a result of diseases affecting the central nervous system (CNS) [3].

Besides the differences in its etiology, nOH also differs clinically (Table 8.1). Especially in neurodegenerative diseases that affect CNS, decrease in diastolic and systolic blood pressure can be profound and progressive enough to prevent a person from standing up. In addition, the profoundness of the drop in blood pressure and

N. Erken · A. T. Isik (✉)
Department of Geriatric Medicine, Faculty of Medicine, Dokuz Eylul University, Izmir, Turkey

© Springer Nature Switzerland AG 2021
A. T. Isik, P. Soysal (eds.), *Orthostatic Hypotension in Older Adults*, https://doi.org/10.1007/978-3-030-62493-4_8

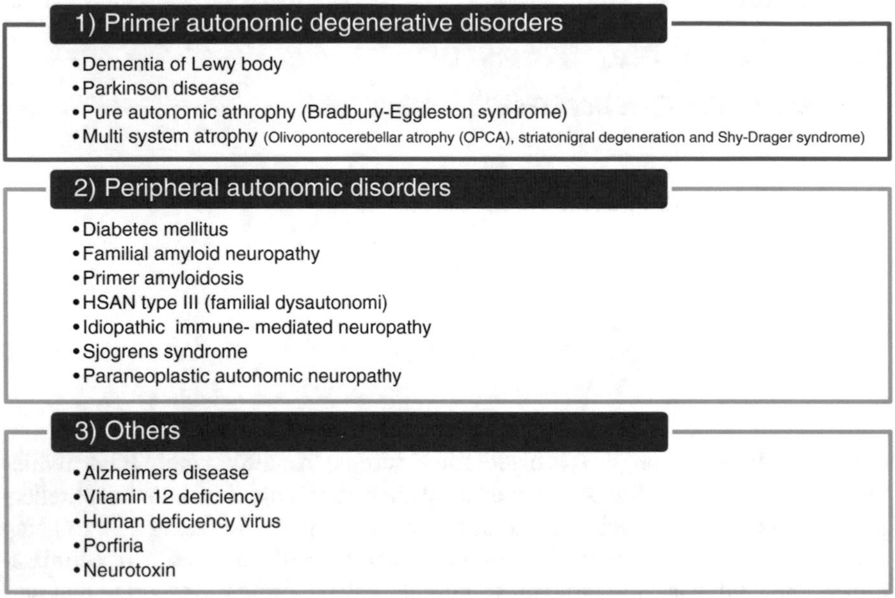

```
┌─────────────────────────────────────────────────────────────────────┐
│  ┌─ 1) Primer autonomic degenerative disorders ──┐                   │
│                                                                       │
│    • Dementia of Lewy body                                            │
│    • Parkinson disease                                                │
│    • Pure autonomic athrophy (Bradbury-Eggleston syndrome)            │
│    • Multi system atrophy (Olivopontocerebellar atrophy (OPCA),       │
│      striatonigral degeneration and Shy-Drager syndrome)              │
└─────────────────────────────────────────────────────────────────────┘
```

```
┌─────────────────────────────────────────────────────────────────────┐
│  ┌─ 2) Peripheral autonomic disorders ──┐                            │
│                                                                       │
│    • Diabetes mellitus                                                │
│    • Familial amyloid neuropathy                                      │
│    • Primer amyloidosis                                               │
│    • HSAN type III (familial dysautonomi)                             │
│    • Idiopathic  immune- mediated neuropathy                          │
│    • Sjogrens syndrome                                                │
│    • Paraneoplastic autonomic neuropathy                              │
└─────────────────────────────────────────────────────────────────────┘
```

```
┌─────────────────────────────────────────────────────────────────────┐
│  ┌─ 3) Others ──┐                                                     │
│                                                                       │
│    • Alzheimers disease                                               │
│    • Vitamin 12 deficiency                                            │
│    • Human deficiency virus                                           │
│    • Porfiria                                                         │
│    • Neurotoxin                                                       │
└─────────────────────────────────────────────────────────────────────┘
```

Fig. 8.1 Etiology of neurogenic orthostatic hypotension [3]*

Table 8.1 Features of neurogenic and non-neurogenic orthostatic hypotension

	Neurogenic	Non-neurogenic
Frequency	Rare	Usual
Onset of disease	Chronic	Acute
Etiology	Neurodegeneration	Dehydration, anemia, etc.
Sympathetic Tonus	Decrease or none	Increase
Level of plasma NE	Up to twofold increase from baseline or none	At least twofold increase from baseline
Tachycardia	Mild or none	Severe
Treatment	Palliative treatment	Triggering disease treatment
Prognosis	Malign	Benign

NE norepinephrine

which stage of the disease it has started, plays an important role in the recognition of the underlying disease.

Pathologies involved in the development of nOH concomitant neurodegenerative diseases [4–6]:

• Releasing decreased norepinephrine by post-ganglionic sympathetic neurons
• Locus cereleus, cerebral neocortex, brainstem degeneration taking part in autonomic nervous system
• The pathology of insular cortex which is the equivalent of baroreceptors in the central nervous system

nOH accounts for less than 10% of all OH cases [7]. However, it should be well known because it is important for the diagnosis and management of various neuro-degenerative diseases (Fig. 8.1). In the rest of the article, nOH etiologies will be mentioned, respectively.

8.1 Primer Autonomic Degenerative Disorders

Diseases affecting CNS include neurodegenerative diseases that result from the accumulation of abnormal protein structures in different parts of the brain, leading to autonomic dysfunction. Dementia of Lewy body (DLB), Parkinson disease (PD), multi system atrophy (MSA), and pure autonomic failure (PAF) are in this group [8]. They can each cause a different rate of autonomic dysfunction and nOH. For example, while in PD the rate of nOH is 20–50%, it can be seen as 30–70% in LBD, 80% in MSA and 100% in PAF [9].

8.1.1 Synucleopathies

α-synuclein which is found in synaptic terminal ends and neuronal cytoplasm [10], is a highly conserved, unfolded protein of 140 amino acids with unknown physiological function. Synucleinopathy takes its name from the intracytoplasmic located Lewy bodies (α-synuclein, ubiquitin and related enzymes), the proteins that cause abnormal phosphorous inflammatory response [8]. It is reflected in the clinic as a neurodegenerative process in which peripheral, autonomic, brainstem, basal ganglia and cortical neurons are affected. The causes of the accumulation of the determinant in neurons (PD, PAF) or glial cells (MSA) or autonomic (PAF) or striatonigral neurons (PD, MSA) are unknown [11]. However, it appears with different clinical presentations that do not always have a clear distinction from each other, depending on the place of accumulation (Table 8.2). In PD and PAF, Lewy body deposits

Table 8.2 Clinical findings of synucleinopathies

	Motor and nonmotor dysfunction	Autonomic dysfunction
PD	Tremor, bradykinesia, rigidity, and postural instability, RSBD, dementia (in late stages)	Later in clinical course
DLB	Tremor, bradykinesia, rigidity, postural instability, dementia, RSBD	Early in clinical course
PAF	None	Diagnose with progressive autonomic dysfunction
MSA	MSA-p: tremor, bradykinesia, rigidity, and postural instability MSA-c: gait ataxia with cerebellar dysarthria, stridor, limb ataxia oroculomotor dysfunction, dystonia, RSBD, dementia	Severe autonomic dysfunction develops early in clinical course

DLB dementia of Lewy body, *MSA-c* multi system atrophy with predominant cerebellum, *MSA-p* multi system atrophy with predominant Parkinsonism, *PD* Parkinson disease, *PAF* pure autonomic failure, *RSBD* rapid eye movement sleep behavior disorder accumulate in the neuronal pericardia and axons Lewy neurites [9]. In MSA, α-synuclein deposits show accumulationin oligodendrocytes [9]. Progression of the neurodegeneration is slow in other diseases except MSA, a rare but progressive disease [12].

8.1.1.1 Parkinson Disease (PD)

PD is a chronic, progressive disease that occurs as a result of degeneration of dopaminergic neurons in the brain and responds dramatically to dopaminergic therapy. Bradykinesia, resting tremor, rigidity and postural instability are observed in the clinic [13]. For this reason, patients generally apply to the clinic due to limitation-slowing of motor function. The disease is evaluated according to the clinical criteria determined by the Movement Disorder Society (MDS) [13]. In addition to movement disorders, autonomic insufficiency usually occurs late in PD, but there is also a subgroup with clinically significant autonomic insufficiency at the beginning of the disease [14]. The presence of OH in PD leads to an increase especially in dementia, fall, and postural instability and has a strong relationship with survival.

8.1.1.2 Dementia of Lewy Body (DLB)

DLB is the most common cause of neurodegenerative dementia after Alzheimer's disease. In addition to the dementia, clinical fluctuation, recurrent visual hallucination, Parkinsonism, dysautonomia, sleep disorders, and neuroleptic sensitivity are observed. Impairment in attention, executive functions and visuospatial perception is prominent in early stage of the disease, while memory is generally affected laterin the course of disease [15]. In order to diagnose probable DLB according to core clinical criteria, in addition to dementia, there must be at least two of them: cognitive fluctuation, visual hallucination, rapid eye movement sleep behavior disorder (RSBD), and Parkinsonism [15]. Parkinsonian symptoms, which can be seen in 70–90% of LBD cases and occur after memory affection, include bradykinesia–akinesia, rigidity, gait disturbance. Although there are studies showing otherwise, rigidity is generally bilaterally symmetrical and milder than PD [16]. Autonomic dysfunction in the course of the disease usually occurs after cognitive impairment, but it should be remembered that it can be observed without any significant signs of cognitive deficiency or parkinsonism [17]. Autonomic dysfunction can be reflected to the clinic as orthostatic hypotension and neuro-cardiovascular instability. In addition, it can lead to urinary incontinence—retention, impotence, constipation, and other gastrointestinal symptoms. Autonomic dysfunction caused by DLB is more serious than PD but expected to be milder than MSA [18].

8.1.1.3 Pure Autonomic Failure (PAF)

It is a neurodegenerative disease defined by Bradbury–Eggleston, with no motor deficits, progressing with isolated autonomic dysfunction, developing sporadically and progressively especially in the sixth decade, usually in men. nOH is a characteristic finding of PAF; however, it may also include supine hypertension, genitourinary dysfunction, constipation or intestinal pseudo obstruction, thermoregulatory dysfunction, anosmia, rapid eye movement sleep behavior disorder, neurologic

Table 8.3 Clinical features of pure autonomic failure

Neurologic	Rigidity, hyperreflexia
Sleep	Rapid eye movement sleep behavior disorder
Cardiovascular	Hypertension, supine hypertension, left ventricular hypertrophy, orthostatic hypotension, postprandial hypotension, syncope
Gastrointestinal	Constipation, obstipation
Extremities	Venous pooling, acral color changes
Thermoregulation	Anhidrosis, compensatory hyperhidrosis
Renal	Renal failure, proteinuria
Hematologic	Anemia
Genitourinary	Urgency, nocturia, urinary retention, incontinence
Sexual	Sexual dysfunction, impotence

symptoms and many systemic involvements including anemia, proteinuria, left ventricular hypertrophy (Table 8.3) [19]. Additionally, when supine hypertension is present (systolic BP greater than or equal to 140 mmHg or diastolic BP greater than or equal to 90 mmHg), it is more appropriate to define OH as a drop of 30 mmHg or greater in systolic BP [19, 20].

α-synuclein is a nonmotor synucleinopathy with positive peripheral autonomic neuronal degeneration, Lewy body-like inclusion bodies in sympathetic ganglion, and common α-synuclein deposits in autonomic neurons. As a result, there is norepinephrine (NE) production and oscillation defect in the peripheral autonomic nervous system [17]. It is important to demonstrate the presence of deep OH during diagnosis, unlike other synucleinopathies. In addition, nausea, sweating or increased temperature during OH are not seen in these patients. Temperature intolerance, sweating, constipation, dry mouth and urinary retention accompany the clinic picture, mostly due to diffuse autonomic insufficiency [21]. These cases with pure autonomic dysfunctions become bed-dependent due to OH in the future. The main cause of mortality is from complications associated with falling. PAF may show a slow progressive course for decades. However, nearly 35% of the patients with PAF have been reported to meet the diagnostic criteria for a synucleinopathy, within 4 years of follow-up [12].

8.1.1.4 Multi System Atrophy (MSA)

Multi System Atrophy is a sporadic disease first described in 1969, accompanied by various combinations of Parkinsonism, cerebellar, pyramidal, autonomic and urological dysfunction. It shows an incidence of 3/100,000 per year [22]. The age of diagnosis is usually fifth decade and is more common in men. The reason is unknown. However, degeneration of myelin in MSA is characteristic. It is thought that the abnormal α-synuclein protein accumulation in oligodendrocytes leads to glial and myelin dysfunction leading to neurodegeneration [23].

According to the results of a small study group confirmed by magnetic resonance imaging, it was observed that white matter hyperintense of MSA patients was more intense when compared with PD [24].

To be able to diagnose probable MSA, adult-onset, autonomic dysfunction should be progressive (impotence with nOH or urinary incontinence, which shows a decrease of more than ≥30 mmHg in systolic blood pressure or more than ≥15 mmHg in diastolic blood pressure by standing up within 3 min.) and the L-dopa response to parkinsonism/cerebellar symptoms should be insufficient. In addition, hyperreflexia and Babinsky positivity can be accepted as a supportive finding for the diagnosis of MSA [25]. Under the MSA umbrella, there are three syndromes as a result of the predominant clinical features depending on the involvement of certain pathways in the brain [26];

- Striatonigral degeneration was redefined as MSA with predominant parkinsonism (MSA-p),
- Olivopontocerebellar atrophy (OPCA) was redefined MSA with predominant cerebellar ataxia (MSA-c)
- Autonomic failure predominates, the term Shy–Drager syndrome (SDS)

Since motor deficit is the most common in MSA-p patients, these patients are often diagnosed with PD. In 80% of these patients, motor deficits predominate and signs of Parkinsonism with progressive akinesia and postural tremor are at the forefront. In two-thirds of patients, tremor spreads to the elbows, but tremor is less common than PD [27]. In addition, camptocormia, anterocollis, postural instability and falls appear. Especially after the motor findings start, the frequency of falling increases within 3 years [28]. Although parkinsonian findings are in the foreground, complaints are progressive regardless of dopaminergic treatment [29]. MSA-c, gait and extremity ataxia due to cerebellar injury, dysarthria and ocular motor abnormalities (gaze-evoked nystagmus, impaired smooth pursuits with saccadic intrusion, and/or ocular dysmetria) are observed [30, 31]. However, it is usually orthostatic hypotension and associated falls that bring the patient to the doctor. In the later stages of MSA, cerebellar and parkinsonian deficits may merge. A severe cognitive impairment is not generally expected. Dysphagia and dystonia can be seen in both MSA types. According to a comprehensive study, sympathetic dysautonomia is observed in 83% of urinary dysfunction and 75% [32].

Shy–Drager syndrome is also known as orthostatic hypotension syndrome or Shy–McGee–Drager syndrome. The main finding in the disease is dysautonomia symptoms. Orthostatic hypotension, bradycardia, lack of accommodation, sialoporia, tear reduction, gastrointestinal dysmotility and urinary retention can be seen. In its pathology, α-synuclein accumulation, which leads to Nigrostriatal and Olivo-Ponto Cerebellar Atrophy, plays a role. Its diagnosis is difficult, and its prognosis is poor because it causes a wide variety of complaints [33].

Autonomic dysfunction, which occurs as a result of neurodegenerative process, affects the vascular system as well as many other systems. For example, as a result of dysfunction of the detrusor muscle, an increase in postvoiding residues may come to the clinic with urinary incontinence. In addition, libido loss and impotence are among the common clinical reflections such as incontinence. In the intestinal system, a decrease in motility may involve different clinical consequences, from simple constipation to Ogilvie's syndrome, a pseudoobstruction, or toxic megacolon [34]. Addition to, postprandial hypotension and disruption in thermoregulation are the outcomes of autonomic dysfunction.

8.1.2 Drugs

Medications can also lead to an increase in the frequency of OH in the elderly. While antihypertensive agents rank first among these drugs, OH may also develop due to the drugs used in the treatment of common neurological and psychiatric diseases in these cases. As a result of the pharmacokinetic and pharmacodynamics changes that occur with advancing age, the elimination of drugs may be delayed and an increase in bioavailability time may occur. Decrease in parietal cell count, slowing of gastric pH increase, delay in gastrointestinal emptying, decrease in mucosal cell count in the intestinal system, decrease in mesenteric—hepatic-renal blood flow, and increase in fat mass due to decrease in total body fluid and changes in liver enzyme activity are the causes of age-related changes in drug pharmacokinetics [35, 36]. Therefore, prescribed for the treatment of the neurodegenerative diseases, many drugs may aggravate the disease course by developing postural hypotension, thereof they should be used with caution.

These drugs are (Table 8.4) [37]:

- Antiparkinsonian agents (dopamine agonists)
- Antidepressants
- Antipsychotics

Dopamine agonists are agents used alone or in combination with a decarboxylase enzyme inhibitor to treat Parkinson's disease. They cause arterial and venous dilatation as a result of myorelaxant effect on vascular muscle cells via dopamine 1 (D1) receptors, and also lead to diuresis and natriuresis. On dopamine 2 (D2) receptors, noradrenaline release from presynaptic nerve endings affects vascular resistance. A decrease in blood pressure is observed by stimulating both receptors [38].

Conditions such as decreased first-pass elimination of the drug from the liver, decrease in the body distribution of the drug due to the decrease in lean muscle mass with advancing age, and prolongation of the drug to be destroyed in the liver due to

Table 8.4 Drug-induced orthostatic hypotension [37][φ]

Drugs		Frequency	Mechanism
Dopamine Agonists	Levodopa	Usual	Vasodilatation (D1[a] Receptor Activity)
Anti-depressants	Amitriptyline, duloxetine, nortriptyline, trazodone	Common	Vasodilatation
Anti-psychotics	Atypical type	Common	Vasodilatation

[a]*D1* dopamine 1

the decrease in the decarboxylase enzyme activity, increases the risk of drug-related side effects [39]. In addition, with the decline of receptor sensitivities with age, the effectiveness of drugs changes. Therefore, the effectiveness of narcotic and sedative drugs (such as antipsychotic, antidepressant) increases. At the same time, antidepressants and antipsychotics, which are generally lipophilic in nature and whose risk of side effects increase with changes in body distribution, also cause OH by causing peripheral alpha1 receptor blockage. In addition, nitrates used in the treatment of supine hypertension and calcium channel blockers increase peripheral venous pondingas a result of vasodilation and decrease postural hypotension by decreasing cardiac output. Therefore, antihypertensive agents may cause lower blood pressure in the elderly than expected [20].

8.2   Peripheral Autonomic Disorders

Diseases involving the peripheral nervous system without neurodegeneration in the CNS can also cause nOH, of which diabetic neuropathy (diabetic autonomic neuropathy–DAN) is the most common [40]. DAN can affect cardiovascular, urogenital, gastrointestinal, pupillomotor, thermoregulatory and sudomotor systems. Several diabetes-related syndromes cause autonomic dysfunction. The most common of these are: diabetic autonomic neuropathy, prediabetes-related autonomic neuropathy, treatment-related painand autonomic neuropathy, and autonomic neuropathy associated with transient hypoglycemia [40]. Especially in hyperglycemic patients, the neuropathy is among the microvascular complications of diabetes. After orthostasis developing secondary to DAN, diurnal variation of blood pressure disappears, and the frequency of supine hypertension and postprandial hypotension can be observed at night [41].

Familial Amyloid Neuropathy, also known as Transthyretin Familial Amyloid Polyneuropathy (TTR-FAP), is an adult-onset severe hereditary neuropathy found in endemic regions. Sensorimotor can bring about various clinical symptoms according to autonomic dysfunction and organ involvement (heart, eyes, kidney, etc.) [42]. Primary Amyloidosis, on the other hand, results from the conversion of soluble immunoglobulin light chains into highly organized amyloid fibrillary aggregates that can lead to organ dysfunction. It progresses with progressive and irreversible damage [43]. Hereditary sensory and autonomic neuropathy (HSAN Type III or Familial Dysautonomia) is a rare neurological disorder caused by its mutation in the inhibitor of kappa light polypeptide gene enhancer in B cells, kinase complex-associated protein (IKBKAP) gene. The mutation causes a tissue-specific deficiency in IκB kinase complex-associated protein (IKAP), a protein that plays a role in the development and survival of neurons. Patients who are homozygous are often born with multiple lesions affecting the afferent fibers, leading to widespread organ dysfunction and increased mortality. The neurodegenerative features of the disease include progressive optic atrophy and gait—ataxia [44]. Neuropathy (sensory ganglionopathy, painful small fiber neuropathy), and transverse myelitis (independently or related neuromyelitis optica) occurs in approximately 20% of Sjogren's syndrome, also known as dryness syndrome [45].

Paraneoplastic autonomic neuropathy is nerve involvement developing in the course of cancer and associated with the disease. Motor and autonomic nervous system effects due to peripheral neuropathy are frequently seen in the clinic. With CD8-positive cytotoxic T cells, dorsal root ganglia damage due to lymphocytic infiltration can develop secondary to various antibodies, including Anti-Hu, anti-CV2/CRMP-5, and anti-ganglionic acetylcholine receptor antibodies [46]. Apart from these, there is an idiopathic immune-mediated neuropathy group with a rate of 20–30% [47].

8.3   Others

Besides synucleinopathies, the frequency of OH is also high in Alzheimer's dementia (AD) and vascular dementia (VaD), which is also known as the most common cause of neurodegenerative dementia. In a study with 13% OH in elderly individuals, it was shown that VaD was 34%, 34% in AD, 49% in PD, and 52% in LBD [48]. Moreover, in AD, deterioration of the basal cortisol level in body fluids (plasma, urine, cerebrospinal fluid) due to disruption of the hypothalamic-pituitary axis, and cerebral blood flow disruption in the cortical perivascular cholinergic terminals may play a role [6, 49]. Furthermore, subtotal luminal occlusion occurs after hyaline fibrosis in the muscular layer around the structures, which are seen in the course of VaD and have an important role in the supply of cerebral blood flow. After parasympathetic innervation ischemia, acetylcholine (ACh) responses quickly, and after synaptic stimulation it is expected to develop arterial relaxation with the release of vasodilator agents. However, a significant decrease in ACh level can be seen in advanced period, and besides this, neurogenic OH may accompany the clinicafter the development of ischemia in the cortex areas that regulate cardiovascular regulation [50]. It is known that vitamin deficiencies, especially vitamin B12 and folic acid deficiency, may result in nOH by causing peripheral neuropathy [51]. Apart from these, there are peripheral neuropathies developing after toxic (chemotherapeutic agents, alcohol consumption and heavy metals and other environmental or biological toxins), infectious (Lyme disease, HIV, leprosy, hepatitis) [52].

8.4   Treatment of Neurogenic Orthostatic Hypotension

In the treatment of nOH, the goal is not to normalize the blood pressure when standing up, but to protect the patient from the mortality and morbidity caused by low blood pressure and increase the quality of life. Treatment consists of three steps (Fig. 8.2) [53]:

- Reduction of aggressive factors
- Non-pharmacological measures
- Pharmacological measures

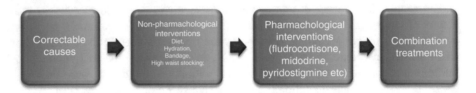

Fig. 8.2 Management of neurogenic orthostatic hypotension

With advanced age, the frequency of comorbid diseases and polypharmacy is observed. In particular, diuretics, alpha blockers, calcium channel blockers, beta blockers, nitrates, tricyclic antidepressants may cause OH or deepen the existing clinic through various mechanisms such as decreased vascular volume, decreased norepinephrine (NE) release in neurovascular junction, vasodilation [53].

In fact, it should be remembered that L-dopa and dopamine agonists used in motor deficit therapy increase OH. Other aggregating and correctable factors are malnutrition, vitamin B12, vitamin D deficiencies, and anemia. Malnutrition is known to cause sarcopenia, fragility, falling, and an increased risk of infection. Even if the relationship between micronutrient insufficiency and OH is not clearly demonstrated, studies reveal the relationship between systolic blood pressure change and malnutrition and/or malnutrition risk [54]. Vitamin D deficiency is known to lead to orthostatic hypotension with decreased renin-angiotensin aldosterone system response, endothelial dysfunction and consequently vasopressor response [55, 56]. In case of vitamin B12 deficiency, vascular resistance is deteriorated as a result of sympathetic system dysfunction as a result of myelinization defect developed in sympathetic post-ganglionic neurons and development of OH becomes easier [57]. With an increase in age and comorbid diseases, absorption defect, poor bone marrow function, erythropoietin failure, as well as intermittent acute or chronic hemorrhage, and anemia are other common correctable problems. Anemia causes a decrease in blood viscosity and oxygen carrying capacity. The reduction of hemoglobin, which also carries nitric oxide (NO), causes an increase in the amount of NO released, leading to a decrease in vasodilation and vascular resistance. In addition, although the underlying mechanism is not clear, it is known that patients have an increase in tolerance to orthostatic symptoms with the use of erythropoietin in the treatment of nOH developing secondary to PAF and MSA [58].

Non-pharmacological methods and patient's education set the cornerstones of OH management. Generally, chronic dehydration is seen in older age. Antihypertensive agents, decreased fluid intake, intervening infections, and caffeine, alcohol and carbohydrate-loaded foods with diuretic effects are factors that precipitate OH [59]. Daily 2–2.5 L fluid intake and an average of 1.5 teaspoons of salt consumption are important. Patients with insufficient salt consumption can use 0.5–1 g salt tablets. Consumption of 500 mL of liquid, which is drunk quickly before getting up in the morning, can raise blood pressure in 5–10 min. However, its effect is maximum 30 min. Sudden movements should be avoided to prevent positional falls. In addition, it is important to prevent constipation caused by autonomic dysfunction and to avoid Valsalva maneuver which reduces intraabdominal pressure of patients [60]. The temperature of the patient's environment is also important. Especially environments with vasodilator effect such as hot shower and sauna should be avoided. Continuity of the prone position is known to impair the blood pressure reflex. However, physical exercises should be done on the back or sitting. It should be remembered that patients with nOH may not tolerate standing exercises. Intra-pool exercises that protect peripheral pressure are ideal exercises, but suddenly leaving the water leads to a sudden decrease in outdoor pressure [61]. It should be remembered that the risk of falling is high in these cases. With eating, splanchnic circulation increases and vasoconstriction develops with the sympathetic system response. However, in patients with autonomic dysfunction, postprandial hypotension is observed, especially within 2 h, due to insufficient reflex response [62]. Preventing venous ponding in the splanchnic area is important in the treatment of OH. Therefore, high waist stocking, including the abdomen and upper leg, support vascular reflex by providing 15–20 mmHg pressure. Isolated abdominal bandages that provide 40 mmHg pressure increase only in the splanchnic area are also among the alternative measures [63].

An important issue to keep in mind about pharmacologic treatment of nOH is supine hypertension (SH), which is common in patients with nOH and may be worsen by drugs used to normalize standing blood pressure. SH is defined as the systolic blood pressure measured in the supine position above 150 mmHg or diastolic blood pressure above 90 mmHg [64]. Therefore, non-pharmacological approaches should be applied first. It is recommended to use pressure bandages throughout the day, to avoid the supine position during the day, to keep the bed head 30°, to consume carbohydrate-rich foods before bedtime and to restrict fluid 1 h before bedtime [65]. In supine hypertension, pharmacological treatment should not be used unless systolic blood pressure is 160–180 mmHg or diastolic 110 mmHg and short-acting agents should be preferred [66].

Angiotensin-converting enzyme (ACE) inhibitors can be used in accordance with the pathophysiology. Short-acting ACEinhibitor (captopril), angiotensin receptor blockers (losartan), calcium channel blockers (nifedipine), hydralazine, minoxidil, glyceryl trinitrate (GTN) patches (must be removed 1 h before getting up) and clonidine are generally recommended in treatment [64–69]. Medical agents should be used with caution in supine hypertension. Some agents may be used in cases where non-pharmacological methods do not work in orthostatic hypotension. In the treatment of nOH, midodrine (α adrenergic agonist), and droxidopa (norepinephrine precursor) have FDA approval [70].

Synthetic mineralocorticoid, which reduces volume depletion at the beginning of medical treatment, fludrocortisone can be used, but it should not be forgotten that it causes side effects and SH in the long term. The initial dose is 0.1 mg/day taken in the morning. It is not recommended to use more than 0.2 mg/day due to increased side effects. It is not used for more than a week or two. The most common side effects in the short term are hypokalemia, lower extremities edema, and SH. In the long term, end organ damage due to fibrosis is observed. The prodrug midodrine is the first recommended drug by the FDA to treat nOH. As a result of its activation, it changes into desglymidodrine and shows peripheral selective alpha-1 adrenergic agonistic effect, leading to increased peripheral venous and arterial pressure [70]. It leads to increased systolic and diastolic blood pressure regardless of position. It rapidly undergoes gastrointestinal absorption and reaches peak plasma concentration in 20–40 min. Plasma half-life is 30 min. Its daily dose is between 2.5 and 10 mg, and the maximum dose is 40 mg/day [71]. It is not recommended to use 4–5 h before bedtime due to the pronounced SH side effect, as well as in severe heart failure, uncontrolled hypertension or urinary retention. Pilomotor reaction, itching, supine hypertension, gastrointestinal side effects and urinary retention are common side effects. In addition, anxiety, temperature intolerance and tachycardia may occur with sympathetic discharge [70, 71].

Droxidopa, another FDA approved synthetic amino acid, is a hydroxyl group added to levodopa and acts as a decarboxylated norepinephrine [72]. Although there is a lower risk of SH compared to midodrine, it is recommended to be used 4–5 h before bedtime. The initial dose is 100 mg/day, and it can be titrated up to a maximum of 600 mg/day. Additionally, erythropoietin, caffeine, pyridostigmine, and nonsteroidal anti-inflammatory can be used in persistent symptoms. However, it should not be forgotten that their effectiveness is limited [72].

The diagnosis and treatment of nOH, which is only one of the consequences of autonomic insufficiency caused by neurodegeneration, has an important role in disease management. With the sudden blood pressure imbalances that may occur due to the position and the decrease of cerebral perfusion, the fall may trigger the risk of immobility, intracerebral events or fractures. Adding new morbidities to this group of diseases, which already have a high burden of disease and cannot have curative treatment, causes the target quality of life to decrease. First of all, education of the patients and their relatives is the main target. It should not be forgotten that pharmacological agents have a place in the treatment, if necessary, after non-pharmacological methods.

References

1. Joseph A, et al. Orthostatic hypotension: a review. Nephrol Ther. 2017;13:S55–67.
2. Smit AAJ, et al. Pathophysiological basis of orthostatic hypotension in autonomic failure. J Physiol. 1999;519(1):1–10.
3. Freeman R. Neurogenic orthostatic hypotension. N Engl J Med. 2008;358(6):615–24. *Made as references.
4. Robertson AD, et al. Orthostatic hypotension and dementia incidence: links and implications. Neuropsychiatr Dis Treat. 2019;15:2181.
5. Freeman R, et al. Consensus statement on the definition of orthostatic hypotension, neurally mediated syncope and the postural tachycardia syndrome. Autonom Neurosci Basic Clin. 2011;161(1):46–8.
6. Isik AT, et al. A comparison of the prevalence of orthostatic hypotension between older patients with Alzheimer's Disease, Lewy body dementia, and without dementia. Exp Gerontol. 2019;124:110628.
7. Fedorowski A, Melander O. Syndromes of orthostatic intolerance: a hidden danger. J Intern Med. 2013;273(4):322–35.

8. Kaufmann H, Biaggioni I. Autonomic failure in neurodegenerative disorders. Semin Neurol. 2003;23(4):351–63.
9. Pilotto A, et al. Orthostatic hypotension and REM sleep behaviour disorder: impact on clinical outcomes in α-synucleinopathies. J Neurol Neurosurg Psychiatry. 2019;90(11):1257–63.
10. Uversky VN. Neuropathology, biochemistry, and biophysics of alpha-synuclein aggregation. J Neurochem. 2007;103(1):17–37.
11. Galvin JE, Lee VM-Y, Trojanowski JQ. Synucleinopathies: clinical and pathological implications. Arch Neurol. 2001;58(2):186–90.
12. Palma J-A, Kaufmann H. Treatment of autonomic dysfunction in Parkinson disease and other synucleinopathies. Mov Disord. 2018;33(3):372–90.
13. Postuma RB, et al. MDS clinical diagnostic criteria for Parkinson's disease. Mov Disord. 2015;30(12):1591–601.
14. Beitz JM. Parkinson's disease: a review. Front Biosci. 2014;6:65–74.
15. McKeith IG, et al. Diagnosis and management of dementia with Lewy bodies: fourth consensus report of the DLB Consortium. Neurology. 2017;89(1):88–100.
16. Strong C, et al. Abnormally phosphorylated tau protein in senile dementia of Lewy body type and Alzheimer disease: evidence that the disorders are distinct. Alzheimer Dis Assoc Disord. 1995;9:218.
17. Garland EM, Hooper WB, Robertson D. Pure autonomic failure. In: Handbook of clinical neurology, vol. 117. Amsterdam: Elsevier; 2013. p. 243–57.
18. Thaisetthawatkul P, et al. Autonomic dysfunction in dementia with Lewy bodies. Neurology. 2004;62(10):1804–9.
19. Coon EA, Singer W, Low PA. Pure autonomic failure. In: Mayo Clinic Proceedings. Amsterdam: Elsevier; 2019.
20. Fanciulli A, et al. Consensus statement on the definition of neurogenic supine hypertension in cardiovascular autonomic failure by the American Autonomic Society (AAS) and the European Federation of Autonomic Societies (EFAS). Clin Auton Res. 2018;28(4):355–62.
21. Singer W, et al. Pure autonomic failure: predictors of conversion to clinical CNS involvement. Neurology. 2017;88(12):1129–36.
22. Papp MI, Kahn JE, Lantos PL. Glial cytoplasmic inclusions in the CNS of patients with multiple system atrophy (striatonigral degeneration, olivopontocerebellar atrophy and Shy-Drager syndrome). J Neurol Sci. 1989;94(1-3):79–100.
23. Jellinger KA. Neuropathology of multiple system atrophy: new thoughts about pathogenesis. Mov Disord. 2014;29(14):1720–41.
24. Umoto M, et al. White matter hyperintensities in patients with multiple system atrophy. Parkinsonism Relat Disord. 2012;18(1):17–20.
25. Khan S, et al. Multiple system atrophy mimicked by multi-organ pathology. Pract Neurol. 2019;19(4):350–1.
26. Gilman S, et al. Consensus statement on the diagnosis of multiple system atrophy. J Neurol Sci. 1999;163(1):94–8.
27. Geser F, et al. The European multiple system atrophy-study group (EMSA-SG). J Neural Transm. 2005;112(12):1677–86.
28. Wenning GK, et al. Multiple system atrophy. Lancet Neurol. 2004;3(2):93–103.
29. Watanabe H, et al. Progression and prognosis in multiple system atrophy: an analysis of 230 Japanese patients. Brain. 2002;125(5):1070–83.
30. Palma J-A, Norcliffe-Kaufmann L, Kaufmann H. Diagnosis of multiple system atrophy. Auton Neurosci. 2018;211:15–25.
31. Krishnan M, et al. Hot cross bun sign–multisystem atrophy (cerebellar type). J Assoc Physicians India. 2018;66(5):87.
32. Köllensperger M, et al. Presentation, diagnosis, and management of multiple system atrophy in Europe: final analysis of the European multiple system atrophy registry. Mov Disord. 2010;25(15):2604–12.
33. Dusejovska M, et al. Shy-Drager syndrome. Cas Lek Cesk. 2010;149(5):225–8.

34. Isik AT, et al. Ogilvie's syndrome in an elderly patient with multi-system atrophy. Clin Auton Res. 2013;23(3):155–6.
35. Zaleon CR, Guthrie SK. Antipsychotic drug use in older adults. Am J Health Syst Pharm. 1994;51(23):2917–43.
36. Kapoor WN. Syncope in older persons. J Am Geriatr Soc. 1994;42(4):426–36.
37. Schoenberger JA. Drug-induced orthostatic hypotension. Drug Saf. 1991;6(6):402–7. ᵠMade as references.
38. Murphy MB. Dopamine: a role in the pathogenesis and treatment of hypertension. J Hum Hypertens. 2000;14(1):S47–50.
39. Verhaeverbeke I, Mets T. Drug-induced orthostatic hypotension in the elderly. Drug Saf. 1997;17(2):105–18.
40. Freeman R. Diabetic autonomic neuropathy. In: Handbook of clinical neurology, vol. 126. Amsterdam: Elsevier; 2014. p. 63–79.
41. Vinik AI, et al. Diabetic autonomic neuropathy. Diabetes Care. 2003;26(5):1553–79.
42. Adams D, et al. The course and prognostic factors of familial amyloid polyneuropathy after liver transplantation. Brain. 2000;123(7):1495–504.
43. Merlini G, et al. Systemic immunoglobulin light chain amyloidosis. NatRrev Dis Prim. 2018;4(1):1–19.
44. Norcliffe-Kaufmann L, Slaugenhaupt SA, Kaufmann H. Familial dysautonomia: history, genotype, phenotype and translational research. Prog Neurobiol. 2017;152:131–48.
45. Berkowitz AL, Samuels MA. The neurology of Sjögren's syndrome and the rheumatology of peripheral neuropathy and myelitis. Pract Neurol. 2014;14(1):14–22.
46. Koike H, Tanaka F, Sobue G. Paraneoplastic neuropathy: wide-ranging clinicopathological manifestations. Curr Opin Neurol. 2011;24(5):504–10.
47. Farhad K, et al. Causes of neuropathy in patients referred as "idiopathic neuropathy". Muscle Nerve. 2016;53(6):856–61.
48. Freidenberg DL, et al. Orthostatic hypotension in patients with dementia: clinical features and response to treatment. Cogn Behav Neurol. 2013;26(3):105–20.
49. Siennicki-Lantz A, Lilja B, Elmståhl S. Orthostatic hypotension in Alzheimer's disease: result or cause of brain dysfunction? Aging Clin Exp Res. 1999;11(3):155–60.
50. Moretti R, et al. Risk factors for vascular dementia: hypotension as a key point. Vasc Health Risk Manag. 2008;4(2):395.
51. Yang G-T, et al. Correlation between serum vitamin B12 level and peripheral neuropathy in atrophic gastritis. World J Gastroenterol. 2018;24(12):1343.
52. Katona I, Weis J. Diseases of the peripheral nerves. In: Handbook of clinical Neurology, vol. 145. Amsterdam: Elsevier; 2018. p. 453–74.
53. Press Y, Punchik B, Freud T. Orthostatic hypotension and drug therapy in patients at an outpatient comprehensive geriatric assessment unit. J Hypertens. 2016;34(2):351–8.
54. Kocyigit SE, et al. Malnutrition and malnutrition risk can be associated with systolic orthostatic hypotension in older adults. J Nutr Health Aging. 2018;22(8):928–33.
55. Li YC, et al. 1,25-Dihydroxyvitamin D 3 is a negative endocrine regulator of the renin-angiotensin system. J Clin Invest. 2002;110(2):229–38.
56. McCarroll KG, et al. Vitamin D and orthostatic hypotension. Age Ageing. 2012;41(6):810–3.
57. Moore A, et al. Orthostatic tolerance in older patients with vitamin B12 deficiency before and after vitamin B12 replacement. Clin Auton Res. 2004;14(2):67–71.
58. Perera R, Isola L, Kaufmann H. Effect of recombinant erythropoietin on anemia and orthostatic hypotension in primary autonomic failure. Clin Auton Res. 1995;5(4):211–3.
59. Brignole M, et al. Practical Instructions for the 2018 ESC Guidelines for the diagnosis and management of syncope. Eur Heart J. 2018;39(21):e43–80.
60. Pavy-Le Traon A. How to manage a patient with orthostatic hypotension. Teaching course 13. In: Proceedings of the 3rd Congress of the European Academy of Neurology; 2017.
61. Palma J-A, Kaufmann H. Epidemiology, diagnosis, and management of neurogenic orthostatic hypotension. Mov Disord Clin Pract. 2017;4(3):298–308.

62. Trahair LG, Horowitz M, Jones KL. Postprandial hypotension: a systematic review. J Am Med Dir Assoc. 2014;15(6):394–409.
63. Arnold AC, Raj SR. Orthostatic hypotension: a practical approach to investigation and management. Can J Cardiol. 2017;33(12):1725–8.
64. Gibbons CH, et al. The recommendations of a consensus panel for the screening, diagnosis, and treatment of neurogenic orthostatic hypotension and associated supine hypertension. J Neurol. 2017;264(8):1567–82.
65. Chisholm P, Anpalahan M. Orthostatic hypotension: pathophysiology, assessment, treatment and the paradox of supine hypertension. Intern Med J. 2017;47(4):370–9.
66. Izcovich A, et al. Midodrine for orthostatic hypotension and recurrent reflex syncope: a systematic review. Neurology. 2014;83(13):1170–7.
67. Arnold AC, et al. Angiotensin II, independent of plasma renin activity, contributes to the hypertension of autonomic failure. Hypertension. 2013;61(3):701–6.
68. Jordan J, et al. Contrasting effects of vasodilators on blood pressure and sodium balance in the hypertension of autonomic failure. J Am Soc Nephrol. 1999;10(1):35–42.
69. Shannon J, et al. The hypertension of autonomic failure and its treatment. Hypertension. 1997;30(5):1062–7.
70. Byun J-I, et al. Efficacy of single or combined midodrine and pyridostigmine in orthostatic hypotension. Neurology. 2017;89(10):1078–86.
71. Freeman R, Landsberg L. The treatment of orthostatic hypotension with dihydroxyphenylserine. Clin Neuropharmacol. 1991;14(4):296–304.
72. Chen JJ, et al. Standing and supine blood pressure outcomes associated with droxidopa and midodrine in patients with neurogenic orthostatic hypotension: a Bayesian meta-analysis and mixed treatment comparison of randomized trials. Ann Pharmacother. 2018;52(12):1182–94.

Orthostatic Hypotension and Complications

9

Nicola Veronese and Jacopo Demurtas

9.1 Introduction

Orthostatic hypotension (OH) is often defined as a sudden drop of at least 20 mmHg in systolic blood pressure (SBP) and/or 10 mmHg in diastolic BP (DBP) upon the change in position (from sitting to standing) [1]. This definition is widely accepted across the world [1].

The prevalence of OH exponentially increases with age and is estimated to be about 10–30% in older adults [2].

A question of utmost importance is that OH should be early detected in older people, and, in this chapter, we will try to report the most important consequences and complications associated with OH, reassumed in Fig. 9.1.

9.2 Association Between Orthostatic Hypotension and Syncope and Falls

The possible association between OH and falls is of great interest in geriatric medicine. Falls are common and associated with several negative outcomes in older populations, such as fractures and disability [3]. In this sense, it is estimated that about one-third of older people fall every year [4], but falls are usually underreported [5].

N. Veronese (✉)
Geriatric Unit, Department of Internal Medicine and Geriatrics, University of Palermo, Palermo, Italy

J. Demurtas
Clinical and Experimental Medicine PhD Program, University of Modena and Reggio Emilia, Modena, Italy

Primary Care Department, USL Toscana Sud Est-Grosseto, Arezzo, Italy

© Springer Nature Switzerland AG 2021
A. T. Isik, P. Soysal (eds.), *Orthostatic Hypotension in Older Adults*,
https://doi.org/10.1007/978-3-030-62493-4_9

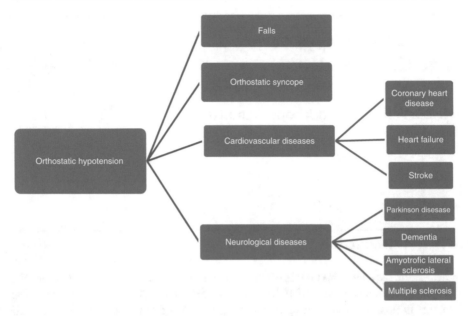

Fig. 9.1 Possible complications of orthostatic hypotension

The association between OH and falls, from an epidemiological perspective, is really complex and still debated. For example, a large meta-analysis published in 2017 and using individual participant data found an increased risk of incident falls in people having OH at the baseline, even if the authors themselves reported some methodological discrepancies [6]. In this sense, other studies failed to find a significant association between OH and risk of falls [7]. In one recent umbrella review regarding the consequences of OH made by our team, we found a significant association between OH and falls, but only of grade III (suggestive) that in practical way means that this association is less significant than expected [8]. Briefly, there are several possible mechanism explaining the possible association between OH and falls. First, OH may cause an acute drop in cerebral oxygenation finally resulting in an impaired cerebral autoregulation, dizziness, and falls [9]. Second, OH might cause brain atrophy, microbleeds, and white matter brain lesions that are strongly associated with falls in epidemiological studies [10]. One interesting study found that OH might also cause falls impairing muscle microcirculation, with a transitory muscle ischemia [11].

Syncope due to OH, often called orthostatic syncope, is another possible complication of OH [12]. After excluding the most dangerous and important causes of syncope, we believe that the history and physical examination are essential components in the evaluation of a patient with orthostatic syncope. It is extremely common to find hypovolemia due to dehydration (e.g., vomiting, diarrhea, fever, or decreased oral intake). Another common risk factor for orthostatic syncope is to stay in stand position after a long period of bedridden, such as hospitalization. Finally, the review of the patients' medication list may often report polypharmacy with a not appropriate use of diuretics, vasodilators, or, less commonly, other antihypertensives, thus requiring withdrawal or dosage correction [13].

9.3 Association Between Orthostatic Hypotension and Cardiovascular Disease

The possible association between OH and cardiovascular disease (CVD) is another topic of great interest since CVDs are the most common causes of death in Western countries. Several epidemiological studies have tried to explore the association between OH and CVD, total and specific.

One of the first studies to explore the possible association between OH and coronary heart disease (CHD) was the study of Rose et al. in 2000 [14]. This study found that in people with OH at the baseline, over 6 years of follow-up, experienced a significant higher risk of CHD than those without this condition of about 85% [14]. In a most recent meta-analysis [15] published in 2016 regarding this topic, the authors found that, over 158,446 participants initially included, OH was associated with a significant risk of about 32% of having CHD during follow-up period. A similar evidence, also in terms of strength, is present for heart failure (HF). In this sense, another meta-analysis found that the presence of OH was associated a higher risk of incident HF in four different cohort studies and in 51,270 participants [16]. Again, the estimated risk was of 30%. Of importance, Xin et al. in their analysis [16] reported that a significant association between OH and HF is particularly strong in middle-age subjects and those with hypertension and diabetes mellitus at baseline [16]. These results highlight the role of OH for incident HF in both the low-risk population and the high-risk population, having known HF risk factors such as diabetes and hypertension. Finally, some research should be done regarding OH and stroke. In a seminal paper, published 20 years ago, the authors report in more than 11,000 participants that OH was associated with a doubled risk of having (ischemic) stroke during follow-up [17]. Most recent works, similarly for the association between OH and HF, have confirmed this association from an epidemiological point of view, but reducing the strength between OH and stroke [15]. However, it should be also reported that OH often appears after a stroke event and OH may complicate the rehabilitation process in these patients [18].

Several hypotheses are useful in trying to explain the association between OH and increased CVD risk. Firstly, patients with OH seem to have increased BP variability related to standing. As a consequence, a large proportion of thoracic blood volume may be placed to lower limbs due to gravity during orthostatism [19]. Therefore, both transitory heart and brain ischemia are supposed to occur as a result of OH [19]. In this sense, acute changes of hemodynamic and organ perfusion status might further trigger a CHD or stroke event. Second, it has been recently reported that OH is often associated with markers of subclinical CVD, such as higher arterial stiffness [20] and activated systematic inflammation [21], which have both been strongly involved in the pathogenesis of atherosclerosis, finally leading to CVD [21, 22].

9.4   Association Between Orthostatic Hypotension and Neurological Conditions

OH is a common complication of several neurological diseases, from multiple sclerosis [23] to amyotrophic lateral sclerosis [24]. However, if OH can be considered a risk factor for neurological conditions is still poorly known, except in the case of stroke (discussed before) and dementia. The typical example is Parkinson's disease (PD). Non-motor aspects of PD are now thought to be relevant. Among them, abnormalities in blood pressure regulation are very common. As much as 40% of PD patients, in fact, report OH, which is a range of conditions, from lightheadedness to falls with serious trauma [25].

Overall, suggestive evidence was found for an association between OH and dementia [8], even if the association was not confirmed taking vascular dementia or Alzheimer's disease as singular entities. The most frequently proposed pathway associating OH to a higher risk of dementia is the recurrent transient brain hypoperfusion hypothesis. Previous literature has in fact reported that cerebral blood flow is decreased in OH [26]. Moreover, decreased brain perfusion during OH was shown by the method of single-photon emission computed tomography [27]. Cerebral hypoperfusion may lead to leukoaraiosis that is underlying neurodegeneration process in dementia [28]. Literature however reports that OH may be detrimental only if compensatory mechanisms are poorly adequate. When cerebral autoregulation is impaired, it poorly reacts for compensating for a drop in cerebral perfusion pressure and fails in maintaining sufficient cerebral blood flow which ultimately might cause ischemic cerebral damage [29]. However, one study reported that no significant association was found between OH and cognitive impairment related with leukoaraiosis, subtle brain microstructural damage, or cerebral blood flow [30]. Finally, it should be recognized that both OH and cognitive function are complicated and affected by multiple factors, practically being multifactorial conditions. Some medical conditions (such as diabetes, alpha-synucleinopathies, and sarcoidosis) are common causes for autonomic neuropathy, and OH is highly prevalent among these diseases [31, 32].

9.5   Association Between Orthostatic Hypotension and Mortality

OH may increase the mortality through the increase of the medical conditions reported before.

From an epidemiological perspective, OH is associated with an increased risk of death, even if this association seems to be mainly driven by concomitant factors [33].

OH often is a condition of impaired hemodynamic homeostasis, in which compensatory neuroendocrine mechanisms are sometimes activated. These mechanisms might increase the trigger of the activation of other biologic effectors, such as platelets or the coagulation cascade. This can further promote the occurrence of cardio/cerebrovascular episodes that can contribute to a higher mortality risk [8].

Moreover, wide swings in blood pressure and supine hypertension associated with OH may provoke intermittent ischemic bouts and increased afterload, finally promoting a permanent end-organ damage, such as left ventricular hypertrophy and decreased renal function [33, 34]. Finally, baroreflex dysfunction, a marker of autonomic nervous system imbalance implicated in the pathogenesis of OH, is mainly characterized by enhanced sympathetic activity and withdrawal of parasympathetic control. This seems to be an important mediator of increased cardiovascular morbidity and mortality [35–37].

9.6   Conclusions

OH is associated with several negative outcomes in older people, including cardiovascular, neurological, and finally higher risk of mortality. These findings stress the importance to assess OH in our daily clinical practice for early finding people that can be managed for improving this condition.

References

1. The American Autonomic Society, The American Academy of Neurology. Consensus statement on the definition of orthostatic hypotension, pure autonomic failure, and multiple system atrophy. The Consensus Committee of the American Autonomic Society and the American Academy of Neurology. Neurology. 1996;46(5):1470.
2. Low PA. Prevalence of orthostatic hypotension. Clin Auton Res. 2008;18(1):8–13.
3. Inouye SK, Brown CJ, Tinetti ME. Medicare nonpayment, hospital falls, and unintended consequences. N Engl J Med. 2009;360(23):2390.
4. Centers for Disease Control and Prevention. WISQARS™ (Web-based Injury Statistics Query and Reporting System). Atlanta, GA: CDC; 2014.
5. Noble DJ, Pronovost PJ. Underreporting of patient safety incidents reduces health care's ability to quantify and accurately measure harm reduction. J Patient Saf. 2010;6(4):247–50.
6. Hartog LC, Schrijnders D, Landman G, Groenier K, Kleefstra N, Bilo HJ, van Hateren KJJ. Is orthostatic hypotension related to falling? A meta-analysis of individual patient data of prospective observational studies. Age Ageing. 2017;46(4):568–75.
7. Jansen S, Bhangu J, de Rooij S, Daams J, Kenny RA, van der Velde N. The Association of Cardiovascular Disorders and Falls: a systematic review. J Am Med Dir Assoc. 2016;17(3):193–9. https://doi.org/10.1016/j.jamda.2015.08.022.
8. Soysal P, Veronese N, Smith L, Torbahn G, Jackson SE, Yang L, Ungar A, Rivasi G, Rafanelli M, Petrovic M. Orthostatic hypotension and health outcomes: an umbrella review of observational studies. Eur Geriatr Med. 2019;10(6):863–70.
9. Mager DR. Orthostatic hypotension: pathophysiology, problems, and prevention. Home Healthc Nurse. 2012;30(9):525–30. https://doi.org/10.1097/NHH.0b013e31826a6805; quiz 530–2.
10. Aoki M, Tanaka K, Wakaoka T, Kuze B, Hayashi H, Mizuta K, Ito Y. The association between impaired perception of verticality and cerebral white matter lesions in the elderly patients with orthostatic hypotension. J Vestib Res. 2013;23(2):85–93. https://doi.org/10.3233/VES-130479.
11. Humm AM, Bostock H, Troller R, Z'Graggen WJ. Muscle ischaemia in patients with orthostatic hypotension assessed by velocity recovery cycles. J Neurol Neurosurg Psychiatry. 2011;82(12):1394–8. https://doi.org/10.1136/jnnp-2011-300444.

12. Grubb BP. Dysautonomic (orthostatic) syncope. In: Syncope: mechanisms and management. Malden, MA: Blackwell Publishing; 2005. p. 72–91.
13. Ziere G, Dieleman J, Hofman A, Pols HA, Van Der Cammen T, Stricker BC. Polypharmacy and falls in the middle age and elderly population. Br J Clin Pharmacol. 2006;61(2):218–23.
14. Rose KM, Tyroler HA, Nardo CJ, Arnett DK, Light KC, Rosamond W, Sharrett AR, Szklo M. Orthostatic hypotension and the incidence of coronary heart disease: the Atherosclerosis Risk in Communities study. Am J Hypertens. 2000;13(6):571–8.
15. Xin W, Mi S, Lin Z, Wang H, Wei W. Orthostatic hypotension and the risk of incidental cardiovascular diseases: a meta-analysis of prospective cohort studies. Prev Med. 2016;85:90–7.
16. Xin W, Lin Z, Li X. Orthostatic hypotension and the risk of congestive heart failure: a meta-analysis of prospective cohort studies. PLoS One. 2013;8(5):e63169. https://doi.org/10.1371/journal.pone.0063169.
17. Eigenbrodt ML, Rose KM, Couper DJ, Arnett DK, Smith R, Jones D. Orthostatic hypotension as a risk factor for stroke: the atherosclerosis risk in communities (ARIC) study, 1987–1996. Stroke. 2000;31(10):2307–13.
18. Kong K-H, Chuo AM. Incidence and outcome of orthostatic hypotension in stroke patients undergoing rehabilitation. Arch Phys Med Rehabil. 2003;84(4):559–62.
19. Smit AA, Halliwill JR, Low PA, Wieling W. Pathophysiological basis of orthostatic hypotension in autonomic failure. J Physiol. 1999;519(Pt 1):1–10. https://doi.org/10.1111/j.1469-7793.1999.0001o.x.
20. Mattace-Raso FU, van der Cammen TJ, Knetsch AM, van den Meiracker AH, Schalekamp MA, Hofman A, Witteman JC. Arterial stiffness as the candidate underlying mechanism for postural blood pressure changes and orthostatic hypotension in older adults: the Rotterdam Study. J Hypertens. 2006;24(2):339–44. https://doi.org/10.1097/01.hjh.0000202816.25706.64.
21. Fedorowski A, Ostling G, Persson M, Struck J, Engstrom G, Nilsson PM, Hedblad B, Melander O. Orthostatic blood pressure response, carotid intima-media thickness, and plasma fibrinogen in older nondiabetic adults. J Hypertens. 2012;30(3):522–9. https://doi.org/10.1097/HJH.0b013e32834fa860.
22. Fan XH, Wang Y, Sun K, Zhang W, Wang H, Wu H, Zhang H, Zhou X, Hui R. Disorders of orthostatic blood pressure response are associated with cardiovascular disease and target organ damage in hypertensive patients. Am J Hypertens. 2010;23(8):829–37. https://doi.org/10.1038/ajh.2010.76.
23. Brown RT, Polinsky RJ, Lee GK, Deeter JA. Insulin-induced hypotension and neurogenic orthostatic hypotension. Neurology. 1986;36(10):1402.
24. Piccione EA, Sletten DM, Staff NP, Low PA. Autonomic system and amyotrophic lateral sclerosis. Muscle Nerve. 2015;51(5):676–9.
25. Sharabi Y, Goldstein DS. Mechanisms of orthostatic hypotension and supine hypertension in Parkinson disease. J Neurol Sci. 2011;310(1-2):123–8.
26. Elmstahl S, Rosen I. Postural hypotension and EEG variables predict cognitive decline: results from a 5-year follow-up of healthy elderly women. Dement Geriatr Cogn Disord. 1997;8(3):180–7. https://doi.org/10.1159/000106629.
27. Toyry JP, Kuikka JT, Lansimies EA. Regional cerebral perfusion in cardiovascular reflex syncope. Eur J Nucl Med. 1997;24(2):215–8.
28. Brown WR, Thore CR. Review: cerebral microvascular pathology in ageing and neurodegeneration. Neuropathol Appl Neurobiol. 2011;37(1):56–74. https://doi.org/10.1111/j.1365-2990.2010.01139.x.
29. Liu H, Zhang J. Cerebral hypoperfusion and cognitive impairment: the pathogenic role of vascular oxidative stress. Int J Neurosci. 2012;122(9):494–9. https://doi.org/10.3109/00207454.2012.686543.
30. Foster-Dingley JC, Moonen JEF, de Ruijter W, van der Mast RC, van der Grond J. Orthostatic hypotension in older persons is not associated with cognitive functioning, features of cerebral damage or cerebral blood flow. J Hypertens. 2018;36(5):1201–6. https://doi.org/10.1097/HJH.0000000000001681.

31. Lim SY, Lang AE. The nonmotor symptoms of Parkinson's disease--an overview. Mov Disord. 2010;25(Suppl 1):S123–30. https://doi.org/10.1002/mds.22786.
32. Gaspar L, Kruzliak P, Komornikova A, Celecova Z, Krahulec B, Balaz D, Sabaka P, Caprnda M, Kucera M, Rodrigo L, Uehara Y, Dukat A. Orthostatic hypotension in diabetic patients-10-year follow-up study. J Diabetes Complicat. 2016;30(1):67–71. https://doi.org/10.1016/j.jdiacomp.2015.08.020.
33. Xin W, Lin Z, Mi S. Orthostatic hypotension and mortality risk: a meta-analysis of cohort studies. Heart. 2014;100(5):406–13. https://doi.org/10.1136/heartjnl-2013-304121.
34. Robertson D. The pathophysiology and diagnosis of orthostatic hypotension. Clin Auton Res. 2008;18(Suppl 1):2–7. https://doi.org/10.1007/s10286-007-1004-0.
35. Sabbah HN. Baroreflex activation for the treatment of heart failure. Curr Cardiol Rep. 2012;14(3):326–33. https://doi.org/10.1007/s11886-012-0265-y.
36. Schwartz PJ, La Rovere MT. ATRAMI: a mark in the quest for the prognostic value of autonomic markers. Autonomic Tone and Reflexes After Myocardial Infarction. Eur Heart J. 1998;19(11):1593–5. https://doi.org/10.1053/euhj.1998.1292.
37. La Rovere MT, Bigger JT Jr, Marcus FI, Mortara A, Schwartz PJ. Baroreflex sensitivity and heart-rate variability in prediction of total cardiac mortality after myocardial infarction. ATRAMI (Autonomic Tone and Reflexes After Myocardial Infarction) Investigators. Lancet. 1998;351(9101):478–84. https://doi.org/10.1016/s0140-6736(97)11144-8.

Nursing Perspective for Older Patient with Orthostatic Hypotension

10

Burcu Akpinar Soylemez and Bilgehan Ozkaya

Orthostatic hypotension (OH) is a common problem among elderly patients, associated with significant morbidity and mortality. The reported prevalence of OH in community-dwelling older people was 22.2%. It was over and even higher among hospitalized older patients [1–3]. OH has been reported to be associated with poor clinical outcomes in older adults like frailty, cardiovascular mortality, cognitive declines, impaired standing balance, increased falls, and impaired of activities of daily living performance [4–7].

OH is not a disease but a sign. It may be symptomatic or asymptomatic. The common symptoms of OH include lightheadedness, dizziness, visual blurring, palpitations, fatigue, "coat-hanger" pain (neck pain and headache localized in the sub-occipital, posterior cervical, and shoulder region), angina pectoris, presyncope, and syncope; these symptoms can severely impact patients' activities of daily living and increase the likelihood of potentially dangerous falls. Prolonged bed rest and many factors trigger orthostatic hypotension in hospitalized patients. Knowing the causative agents in OH is one of the issues that the nurse should know and pay attention to when planning care for patients at risk [8–10]. Because of their patient contact, nurses can play a key role in identifying and evaluating patients at risk for OH [11].

Asymptomatic patients do not usually require treatment. However, OH should be evaluated carefully, even with minor complaints, even if asymptomatic. OH may be

B. Akpinar Soylemez (✉)
Department of Internal Medicine Nursing, Faculty of Nursing, Dokuz Eylul University, Izmir, Turkey
e-mail: burcu.akpinar@deu.edu.tr

B. Ozkaya
Department of Internal Medicine Nursing, Faculty of Nursing, Dokuz Eylul University, Izmir, Turkey

Department of Internal Medicine Nursing, Institute of Health Sciences, Dokuz Eylul University, Izmir, Turkey
e-mail: bilgehan.ozkaya@deu.edu.tr

© Springer Nature Switzerland AG 2021
A. T. Isik, P. Soysal (eds.), *Orthostatic Hypotension in Older Adults*,
https://doi.org/10.1007/978-3-030-62493-4_10

the first sign of a serious illness. Due to the presence of multiple comorbid conditions and nonspecific signs and symptoms, treatment of orthostatic hypotension in the elderly is often challenging. Instead of aiming to achieve arbitrary blood pressure goals, the treatment of orthostatic hypotension should be directed toward ameliorating symptoms, correcting any underlying cause, improving the patient's functional status, and reducing the risk of complications [8, 12].

Reviews and guidelines for management of OH recommend starting with non-pharmacologic strategies before progressing to pharmacologic strategies if the former prove insufficient. Given that pharmacologic therapies for OH can cause significant cardiovascular side effects, including supine hypertension and ventricular hypertrophy, it is imperative to establish which non-pharmacologic strategies can be recommended to patients for safe and effective management of OH [13, 14].

According to a systematic review evaluating the level of evidence of non-pharmacological interventions for management of OH, there were eight identified non-pharmacologic interventions for management of orthostatic hypotension under two general categories: physical modalities (exercise, functional electrical stimulation, compression, physical countermaneuvers, compression with physical countermaneuvers, sleeping with head up) and dietary measures (water intake, meals). Strong levels of evidence were found for four of the eight interventions: functional electrical stimulation in spinal cord injury, compression of the legs and/or abdomen, physical countermaneuvers in various patient populations, and eating smaller and more frequent meals in chronic autonomic failure. However, it was stated that these results are based on a limited number of studies with small sample size [14].

Treatment for OH in the acute setting starts with addressing the reversible causes of OH. The next step is non-pharmacological interventions, with an emphasis on patient education regarding associated symptoms (presyncope, syncope, and falls) and lifestyle modifications. Patients should be educated on non-pharmacological interventions such as: the importance of hydration, dietary changes, daily physical activity, slow rising, raising the head of the bed during sleeping, leg crossing while standing, the use of compression garments on the abdomen or lower extremities, and physical countermaneuvers that can help manage their symptoms of OH [10, 14, 15].

The aim of nursing care in OH is to determine the risk factors for the elderly and to plan and implement interventions to prevent the possible negative effects and improve the patient's condition. Elderly individuals who are hospitalized and who are in long-term bed rest and who have risk factors that lead to development of OH should be carefully evaluated in hospitals or care institutions. Educations should be planned and implemented in order to carefully evaluate the elderly individuals with OH risk or signs and to make activity plans accordingly. Elderly individuals hospitalized with a diagnosis of OH or staying in a nursing home should be provided with safety precautions to prevent falls. Patient education is crucial in this issue. The patient and formal/informal caregivers should be informed about the causes and management of OH causes. The education plan of the patient should be planned together with the physician, nurse, and physiotherapist. The use of aids to move, muscle stretching exercises, leg position, elevation of the toes, elevation of the legs,

Table 10.1 Non-pharmacologic interventions for the management of OH [11]

Concomitant medications
• Avoid or carefully manage medications (e.g., a-blockers, diuretics) that can cause or worsen symptoms of OH.
Compression garments
• Wear abdominal binders when out of bed.
• Knee-high garments are not sufficient but must be at least thigh-high to be effective (compression: 23–32 mmHg).
Dietary changes
• Adequate hydration: eight glasses of water daily, plus two additional 8 oz (236–250 mL) glasses before prolonged standing.
• Increased salt intake: up to two additional teaspoons daily.
• Avoid carbohydrate-rich meals and alcohol.
"Head-up" rest/sleep position
• Expert clinical opinion: elevate head of the bed 6–9 in. to reduce risk of supine hypertension.
• Avoid fast movements, sudden standing up or standing still for long periods of time.
• Keep your feet in a crossed position while standing.
Low-impact exercise to improve physical conditioning
• Recumbent stationary bike, rowing machine, aquatic exercise.
• Avoid exercises that
– Increase orthostatic stress (e.g., treadmill)
– Increase risk of overheating or occurring in hot environments

tilt training should be done together with the physiotherapist. In addition to the proposed pharmacologic strategies, the education on non-pharmacologic strategies are within the responsibility of the nurse [8, 16, 17]. The non-pharmacological interventions about patient education are given in Table 10.1.

The nursing care interventions that are specific to OH and the training education topics to be given to elderly individuals are given below.

10.1 Evaluate Blood Pressure

It is important to evaluate blood pressure with the right time and method. Orthostatic hypotension can occur at any time of day. However, it is more likely to occur before breakfast in the morning than in the afternoon. Therefore, morning evaluation of orthostatic hypotension is more appropriate [8, 16, 18, 19]. Large differences in the measurement technique may affect the treatment and reporting prevalence of orthostatic hypotension. Accurate blood pressure measurement is also important for assessing falls and cardiovascular risk. Blood pressure measurements made by nurses play an important role in the diagnosis. Therefore, these measurements must be performed correctly [19, 20]. Additionally, as OH may present differently depending on time of day, meals, hydration, and activity level, the consensus panel suggests that patients should also monitor BP and HR at home to create a 1-week BP/HR diary. Patients, their caregivers, or a nurse should measure supine-to-standing BP (or seated-to-standing BP) upon waking (before taking medications), when symptoms occur, and at bedtime [11, 21].

10.2   Education

The aim of intervention in OH is to educate the individual about the risks of OH. Education should be provided, especially if the factors causing orthostatic hypotension can be altered or corrected. Educating the patient and family about the causes, consequences, and symptoms of orthostatic hypotension is very important. Individualized therapy is the key to managing orthostatic hypotension. Collaboration of the patient is necessary for a therapeutic approach. Maintaining communication and compliance is particularly important in individuals with chronic orthostatic hypotension [8, 16, 19, 22].

10.3   Activity/Exercise

Patients should change their position slowly and avoid lie still. It is important to teach patients to gradually change their posture (especially after long-term bed rest). For supine patients, do abdominal and leg muscle strengthening exercises before sitting (crossing the legs several times) and sitting on the side of the bed for a few minutes before getting up, increase cardiac output, and facilitate the return of blood to the heart [8, 18, 23–25]. Exercises such as crunching legs by stretching leg, hip and calf muscles, suppressing splenic vessels by reducing abdominal pressure, and squatting to reduce venous insufficiency have been reported to be effective in temporarily reducing orthostatic hypotension [13]. Blood pressure and pulse should be measured before the patient can stand up, then the measurements (both measurements) should be repeated with the feet hanging down the edge of the bed while sitting on the bed. The patient should be kept in this position for 1–3 min, and blood pressure and pulse should be reevaluated at the end of this period. Symptoms in the patient should also be observed [22, 25].

The time spent sitting down during the day should be increased for long-term bed rest patients. The head of the bed should be raised 10–20° while the patient is asleep. Reclining in this position increases the blood pressure by activating the renin-angiotensin-aldosterone system, providing aldosterone excretion, sodium and water retention [13, 15, 21–23, 25, 26]. Do not stand still for a long time. The venous pressure in the ankle is 85–90 mmHg when the effect of gravity is fully revealed when standing still. The pooling of blood in the leg veins reduces venous return, and as a result, cardiac output sometimes falls to the level of fainting. However, the rhythmic contraction of the leg muscles while the person is standing reduces the venous pressure in the legs to less than 30 mmHg by pushing the blood towards the heart [27]. Strenuous exercises should be avoided and arms should not be worked on the shoulders [22].

Early mobilization and avoidance of physical deconditioning in the acute care setting has a cardinal role in treating and preventing OH in hospitalized older patients. For patients who have been restricted to the bed, physical countermaneuvers, such as changing body position, squatting or leaning forward as opposed to sitting, and encouraging activity can be helpful in preventing and treating OH. Of these maneuvers, the isometric handgrip, in which the patient tenses their arms for 2 min or until the first sign of impending syncope, has shown to improve blood pressure and OH symptoms, especially in patients with neurocardiogenic syncope. Meanwhile, lower body muscle tensing for approximately 40 s after standing from squatting position has also showed to improve BP and symptoms. Simple positional changes can be an easy way to improve OH without using medications in the elderly [15].

The practical approach is for the patient to contract a group of muscles bilaterally for about 30 s, relax, and then repeat the maneuver. Simple maneuvers include standing up on their toes, or crossing their legs and squeezing. Some patients manage to unobtrusively contract their buttocks, thighs, and calves while they stand. These maneuvers result in a transient increase in total peripheral resistance [16].

Patients should be encouraged to do at least the activities of daily living. While prolonged exercises cause orthostatic hypotension, moderate aerobic exercises that are not excessive can help prevent orthostatic hypotension and improve cardiovascular reflexes. However, exercises should be individually controlled and should be discontinued when symptoms occur [8, 19, 28].

Patients should avoid activities and situations that can increase the risk of falling and fainting, such as very hot baths or moving their arms above their head. Warm environments cause an increase in body temperature and vasodilatation of the vessels resulting in a drop in blood pressure. Exercises should be planned individually in accordance with the functional level, general condition, and health status of the elderly individual, and strenuous exercises should be avoided. Bending the waist should be avoided to get anything off the ground or to reach something at the extreme point. Using supportive tools such as walking sticks, walkers, and even bedside tables or chair armrests can reduce the risk of falls and injuries [8, 18, 22, 23]. Patients should also be counseled how to safely improve physical conditioning through low-impact exercise (e.g., recumbent stationary bicycle, aquatic workouts, rowing machine) [11, 21].

10.4   Elastic Bandage

Elastic bandage and pressure/varicose stockings are recommended to be worn all day as it can increase cardiac output and blood pressure while standing by preventing venous accumulation [13, 18, 22, 23, 29].

One study that looked at patients with progressive OH demonstrated a decrease in blood pressure drop with the use of compression bandages ($P = 0.002$) and symptoms relief continued after 1 month of use ($P = 0.001$) [15, 30]. Another study evaluated the effectiveness of high compression leg bandaging in preventing seated postural hypotension (PH) during the initial phase of ambulation, among elderly inpatients without a history of PH. It was compared the occurrence of seated PH between patients who were bandaged and unbandaged. The rate of seated PH was significantly lower in the bandaged than the unbandaged group. It was concluded that during ambulation of elderly inpatients, high compression leg bandaging is beneficial to prevent seated PH [31]. Compression leg bandaging is inexpensive and safe and may be easily applied by healthcare providers to hospitalized patients. Among inpatients at a high risk for development of PH, the use of this technique is recommended as a non-pharmacologic intervention [31].

10.5   Abdominal Binder

Compression of venous capacitance bed reduces venous pooling and orthostatic fall in BP. The largest venous capacitance bed is the splanchnic-mesenteric bed. Hence, compression of this bed by abdominal compression is much more effective than compressing the leg veins because of its low volume. Some stockings are available that compress legs and abdomen, but many patients find the stockings very difficult to apply. A practical alternative is to wear an abdominal binder as a routine. If additional compression is needed, leg stockings are additionally worn [16].

10.6   Diet

Patients should generally eat small meals and avoid standing up suddenly after eating. To prevent the post-meal formation of orthostatic hypotension, low-carbohydrate meals (six small meals instead of three large meals) should be eaten. Large meals may increase peripheral blood vessels and reduce peripheral vascular resistance. Alcohol intake should be avoided because it causes splenic vasodilatation [18, 21]. It is important to increase the daily fluid intake of patients to prevent dehydration. For patients without heart failure and hypertension, daily sodium salt (5–10 mg/day) and water (at least 5–6 cups/day) intake should be increased. Drinking water before meals can reduce post-meal hypotension. Salt and fluid intake should be increased in extreme heat and febrile diseases [18, 23, 25, 26, 28]. Drinking water is thought to increase blood pressure in individuals with normal healthy and orthostatic hypotension and autonomic failure. However, it is stated that the mechanism of water to increase blood pressure is not yet clear and the discussions on this issue continue [25, 32]. It is suggested that water gives good results at least 30 min before getting out of bed and drinking early in the morning and before meals [33].

10.7   Bath Therapy

Bath treatment, especially exposure to cold or heat of the extremities or the whole body, has been suggested to improve circulatory reflexes. In patients with moderate orthostatic hypotension, a change in the temperature of the water from hot to cold several times during a daily shower may improve postural reflexes. The exposure of the body to the cold activates the sympathetic nervous system, leading to an increase in vascular resistance, and thus an increase in blood pressure throughout the body. Patients with moderate orthostatic hypotension can be bathed in a chair. In cases where orthostatic hypotension is more severe, immersion of the patient's arms and legs into a hot/cold tub may help [8, 19, 33].

References

1. Chen L, Xu Y, Chen XJ, Lee WJ, Chen LK. Association between Orthostatic hypotension and frailty in hospitalized older patients: a geriatric syndrome more than a cardiovascular condition. J Nutr Health Aging. 2019;23(4):318–22.
2. Liguori I, Russo G, Coscia V, Aran L, Bulli G, Curcio F, et al. Orthostatic hypotension in the elderly: a marker of clinical frailty? J Am Med Dir Assoc. 2018;19(9):779–85.
3. Saedon NIZ, Pin Tan M, Frith J. The prevalence of orthostatic hypotension: a systematic review and meta-analysis. J Gerontol. 2020;75(1):117–22.
4. Angelousi A, Girerd N, Benetos A, Frimat L, Gautier S, Weryha G, et al. Association between orthostatic hypotension and cardiovascular risk, cerebrovascular risk, cognitive decline and falls as well as overall mortality: a systematic review and metaanalysis. J Hypertens. 2014;32(8):1562–71.
5. Hartog LC, Schrijnders D, Landman GWD, Groenier K, Kleefstra N, Bilo HJG, et al. Is orthostatic hypotension related to falling? A meta-analysis of individual patient data of prospective observational studies. Age Ageing. 2017;46(4):568–75.
6. Iseli R, Nguyen VTV, Sharmin S, Reijnierse EM, Lim WK, Maier AB. Orthostatic hypotension and cognition in older adults: a systematic review and meta-analysis. Exp Gerontol. 2019;120:40–9.
7. Shaw BH, Borrel D, Sabbaghan K, Kum C, Yang Y, Robinovitch SN, et al. Relationships between orthostatic hypotension, frailty, falling and mortality in elderly care home residents. BMC Geriatr. 2019;19(1):80.
8. Karadakovan A. Nursing care in orthostatic hypotension [Ortostatik hipotansiyona hemşirelik bakımı]. In: Soysal P, Işık AT, editors. Geriatric syndromes in geriatric practice [Geriatri pratiğinde geriatrik sendromlar]. İzmir: US Akademi; 2018. p. 411–6.
9. Palma JA, Kaufmann H. Management of orthostatic hypotension. Continuum (Minneap Minn). 2020;26(1):154–77.
10. Tzur I, Izhakian S, Gorelik O. Orthostatic hypotension: definition, classification and evaluation. Blood Press. 2019;28(3):146–56.
11. Biswas D, Karabin B, Turner D. Role of nurses and nurse practitioners in the recognition, diagnosis, and management of neurogenic orthostatic hypotension: a narrative review. J Gen Intern Med. 2019;12:173–84.
12. Gupta V, Lipsitz LA. Orthostatic hypotension in the elderly: diagnosis and treatment. Am J Med. 2007;120(10):841.
13. Lahrmann H, Cortelli P, Hilz M, Mathias CJ, Struhal W, Tassinari M. EFNS guidelines on the diagnosis and management of orthostatic hypotension. Eur J Neurol. 2006;13:930–6.
14. Mills PB, Fung CK, Travlos A, Krassioukov A. Nonpharmacologic management of orthostatic hypotension: a systematic review. Arch Phys Med Rehabil. 2015;96(2):366.
15. Patel K, Kiszko K, Torbati A. Therapeutic advances in the management of orthostatic hypotension. Am J Ther. 2018;25(1)
16. Low PA, Tomalia VA. Orthostatic hypotension: mechanisms, causes, management. J Clin Neurol. 2015;11:220–6.
17. Shibao C, Biaggioni I, Lipsitz LA. ASH position paper: evaluation and treatment of orthostatic hypotension. J Clin Hypertens. 2013;15(3):147–53.

18. Sclater A, Alagiakrishnan K. Orthostatic hypotension: a primary care primer for assessment and treatment. Geriatrics. 2004;59:22–7.
19. Türk G, Eşer İ. Prevention of orthostatic hypotension [Ortostatik hipotansiyonun önlenmesi]. J Cumhuriyet Univ School Nurs [Cumhuriyet Üniversitesi Hemşirelik Yüksek Okulu Dergisi]. 2007;11(1):32–6.
20. Bragg F, Kumar NP. Orthostatic hypotension in an octogenarian - an unusual presentation. Age Ageing. 2005;34:307–9.
21. Gibbons CH, Schmidt P, Biaggioni I, Frazier-Mills C, Freeman R, Isaacson S, et al. The recommendations of a consensus panel for the screening, diagnosis, and treatment of neurogenic orthostatic hypotension and associated supine hypertension. J Neurol. 2017;264(8):1567–82.
22. Pendrak T. Orthostatic hypotension: catching the fall in BP. LPN. 2005;1(5):4–7.
23. Sahni M, Lowenthal DT, Meuleman J. A clinical, physiology and pharmacology evaluation of orthostatic hypotension in the elderly. Int Urol Nephrol. 2005;37:669–74.
24. Smith AAJ, Wieling W, Fujimura J, Denq JC, Opfer-Gehrking TL, Akarriou M, et al. Use of lower compression to combat orthostatic hypotension in patients with autonumic dysfunction. Clin Auton Res. 2004;14:167–75.
25. Türk G, Eşer İ. Effect of standard nursing care on the development of orthostatic hypotension in elderly [Standart Hemşirelik Bakımının Yaşlı Bireylerde Ortostatik Hipotansiyon Gelişimine Etkisi]. J Ege Univ Nurs Fac [Ege Üniversitesi Hemşirelik Fakültesi Dergisi]. 2016;32(2):85–96.
26. Mansoor GA. Orthostatic hypotension due to autonomic disorders in the hypertension clinic. Am J Hypertens. 2006;19:319–26.
27. Ganong WF. Dynamics of blood and lymph flow [Kan ve lenf akımının dinamiği]. In: Turkish Society of Physiological Sciences, translator. Medical physiology [TıbbiFizyoloji]. İstanbul: Nobel TıpKitabevleri. 20th ed.; 2002. p. 556–622.
28. Iwanczyk L, Weintraub NT, Rubenstein LZ. Orthostatic hypotension in the nursing home setting. J Am Med Dir Assoc. 2005;7:163–7.
29. Newton JL, Frith J. The efficacy of nonpharmacologic intervention for orthostatic hypotension associated with aging. Neurology. 2018;91(7):e652–6.
30. Podoleanau C, Maggi R, Brignole M, Croci F, Incze A, Solano A, et al. Lower limb and abdominal compression bandages prevent progressive orthostatic hypotension in elderly persons. J Am Coll Cardiol. 2006;48:1425–32.
31. Papismadov B, Tzur I, Izhakian S, Barchel D, Swarka M, Phatel H, et al. High compression leg bandaging prevents seated postural hypotension among elderly hospitalized patients. Geriatr Nurs. 2019;40(6):558–64.
32. Mathias CJ, Young TM. Water drinking in the management of orthostatic intolerance due to orthostatic hypotension, vasovagal syncope and the postural tachycardia syndrome. Eur J Neurol. 2004;11:613–9.
33. Oldenburg O, Kribben A, Baumgart D, Philipp T, Erbel R, Cohen MV. Treatment of orthostatic hypotension. Curr Opin Pharmacol. 2002;2:740–7.

Prevention and Treatment

11

Banu Buyukaydin and Rumeyza Turan Kazancioglu

Orthostatic hypotension (OH) prevalence increases with age. Along with impaired physical activity, hypertension, diabetes mellitus, renal diseases, Parkinson's disease, specific medications—mainly antihypertensive and antidepressant agents—, and finally polypharmacy are the major risk factors. The presence of OH has been associated with adverse cardiovascular outcomes such as coronary artery disease, atrial fibrillation, heart failure, strokes, and non-cardiovascular problems like cognitive dysfunction, dementia, falls, fractures, and depression [1]. Also, in clinical practice, malnutrition risk and some drugs—alpha-1 blockers, neuroleptics, and memantine—are presented as significant predictors of OH [2]. Preventive measures should contain multidirectional approach containing these comorbidities and risk factors. For providing this perspective, OH must be accepted as a novel therapeutic target for all elderly patients and should be a part of basic clinical evaluation.

The treatment of OH includes non-pharmacological and pharmacological interventions [3]. Improvement of the symptoms and functional status are the major targets. Despite several studies, there is no standardized treatment modality. According to comorbidities and OH severity, treatment options should be determined. The final target of the applied treatment is to improve symptomatology and provide independence for daily activities.

As in all other patient groups, acute OH management initially starts with evaluating the acute medical problems in the elderly. These conditions include volume depletion, acute heart failure, cardiac arrhythmia, stroke, major bleeding, or sepsis. After ruling out these acute problems, the conditions and the medications that may decrease blood pressure or exacerbate OH should be investigated (Tables 11.1 and 11.2). Medication management should be individualized according to comorbidities, frailty, life expectancy, and discontinuation risk for specific drugs. In potentially causative medications, antihypertensive agents, antidepressants, and

B. Buyukaydin (✉) · R. Turan Kazancioglu
Department of Internal Medicine, Bezmialem Vakif University, School of Medicine, Istanbul, Turkey

© Springer Nature Switzerland AG 2021
A. T. Isik, P. Soysal (eds.), *Orthostatic Hypotension in Older Adults*,
https://doi.org/10.1007/978-3-030-62493-4_11

Table 11.1 The events that
may decrease blood pressure
or exacerbate orthostatic
hypotension

• Quickly rising after prolonged sitting or lying down
• Prolonged motion-less standing
• Vigorous physical exertion
• Carbohydrate-heavy meals and alcohol ingestion
• Straining for micturition or defecation
• Heat exposure or fever

Table 11.2 The medications
that may decrease blood
pressure or exacerbate
orthostatic hypotension

Pharmacological class, for example, drugs
Diuretics: Furosemide
Antihypertensive agents: Clonidine, labetalol, verapamil, captopril, hydralazine
Tricyclic antidepressants: Imipramine
Nontricyclic antidepressant: Trazodone, paroxetine, and venlafaxine
Antiparkinsonian agents: Levodopa, bromocriptine ropinirole, and pramipexole
α1-blockers: Tamsulosin
Drugs for prostatism/erectile dysfunction: Prazosin, terazosin, and sildenafil
Monoamine oxidase inhibitors: Phenelzine
Neuroleptics: Chlorpromazine and quetiapine
Autonomic neuropathy inducing drugs: Amiodarone, vincristine, and cisplatin
Narcotics and nitrates: Morphine
Insulin

antiparkinsonian drugs are critical [4]. Discontinuation, dose reduction, or replacement of possible agents are the main procedures. But for antihypertensive medications, this advice should be performed with caution for several reasons. Although the relationship between sympatholytic (e.g., α- and β-adrenergic antagonists) and OH has been established, the relation with other antihypertensive agents with OH is uncertain. Moreover, uncontrolled blood pressure can potentiate OH because of increased pressor diuresis, and it has been related to higher OH rates [5] and increased risk of falls [6]. Modifications of treatment include non-pharmacological interventions, dose lowering of medications, and acceptance of more flexible blood pressure targets in frail patients. Angiotensin-converting enzyme inhibitors, angiotensin receptor blockers, and calcium channel blockers are less likely to lead OH and should be preferred [7].

Non-pharmacological lifestyle interventions can result in a modest (10–15 mmHg) increase in blood pressure. But in many cases, they provide a substantial clinical improvement. Avoidance of triggering factors like rapid standing up, hot environments, large meals, and prolonged supine position are the major advices. For reducing the venous pooling, physical counter maneuvers are recommended. These maneuvers include squatting, standing with legs crossed, tensing of leg muscles, breathing maneuvers, avoiding getting up too rapidly, and avoiding standing motionless. They can help maintain blood pressure during daily activities [8]. Abdominal and lower extremity compression binders reduce venous pooling to improve orthostatic tolerance. They provide a reduction of venous capacitance and an increase in total peripheral resistance when graded pressures of at least 30–40 mmHg [9]. But compression of the legs alone is not usable according to compression of the abdomen because of the small venous capacitance of the calves and thighs compared with that of the splanchnic mesenteric bed. But these garments and stockings are uncomfortable to wear especially in elderly patients with comorbidities.

The avoidance of hypovolemia and providing an increase in the intravascular volume are the other targets for the effectiveness of pharmacological treatments. Adequate water intake (2–3 L/day) and sodium consumption (6–9 g/day) are recommended. The rapid ingestion of 500 mL water (in about 5 min) can provide rising in systolic arterial pressure of 30 mmHg [10]. But many elderly people cannot take in this much, and it can be advised that they take at least one glass of fluid with meals. Sodium intake should be maximized if tolerated, but in patients, who have supine hypertension, uncontrolled hypertension and comorbidities with fluid retention like heart failure, renal, or liver failure caution should be tailored. For increased central volume, the head of the bed should be elevated by 10–20° or 10 cm to decrease nocturnal hypertension and nocturnal diuresis [11].

In terms of lifestyle modifications, patients should be encouraged for exercise as tolerated. As deconditioning from physical activity exacerbates OH [12], training in a supine or sitting position is recommended (e.g., recumbent bicycling or swimming). Also, isotonic exercises (e.g., light weight lifting) should be preferred rather than isometric exercises because of incorrect straining and breath-holding during isometric exercises (e.g., holding weights in the same position) may decrease venous return. The other advice includes eating small frequent meals, avoiding alcohol and situations that increase body temperature such as prolonged hot showers. For the proper control of OH, education is an important factor. The patients should be informed and educated for the conditions (and their mechanisms) that can lower blood pressure. The patients should also be instructed on how to manage this orthostatic decompensation and modify the activities of daily living [8]. Although these non-pharmacological advices often have inefficient compliance, they are cost-effective, safely applied, and usually sufficient in mild diseases. But in moderate and severe diseases, pharmacological approaches should be considered [13].

Pharmacological therapy focuses on increasing blood volume or raising peripheral vascular resistance. Because of this, the presence of hypertension or underlying cardiovascular disease must be considered for each patient. In patients with these comorbidities, short-acting pressor agents to increase vascular resistance are preferred. One of these, *Midodrine* is a short-acting alpha-agonist that reduces the venous pooling in the splanchnic circulation and lower extremities and increases the peripheral vascular resistance. It is effective, especially when used for neurogenic OH. It has been found to increase standing blood pressure and decrease OH symptoms [14]. The starting dose is 5 mg three times per day, but most patients respond 10 mg three times per day. But it was also associated with a sixfold increase risk of supine hypertension [15]. For avoiding this risk, the supine posture for a few hours following each dose or lying down in a head-up position should be advised [16]. The other side effects include piloerection, urinary retention, and scalp paresthesias. In terms of the drug interactions, midodrine can trigger bradycardia, arrhythmias, or atrioventricular (AV) block with beta-blockers or calcium channel blockers. Also, with steroids, it can have an increased hypertensive effect.

Droxidopa (100–600 mg, PO), a synthetic prodrug that is converted into norepinephrine in both central and peripheral nervous system, is another medication for neurogenic OH. Circulating norepinephrine is maximally increased after 6 h with persistent elevation for 46 h. In a recent analysis, it was associated with a 66% reduction in falls [17]. ESC guidelines suggest that further evidence is needed to confirm the efficacy. But American College of Cardiology American Heart Association syncope guidelines recommend droxidopa for syncope due to neurogenic OH with a class IIa indication [18]. In patients with congestive heart failure and chronic renal failure, caution is recommended and side effects include headache, fatigue, nausea, and dizziness.

In patients, without hypertension or heart failure, *Fludrocortisone* is considered. Fludrocortisone promotes sodium and water retention acting at renal mineralocorticoid receptors. The indicated initial dose is 0.1–0.2 mg daily early in the morning. Patients should be monitored for fluid overload, headaches, supine hypertension, and hypokalemia. Also, in patients with heart failure, a higher rate of hospitalizations is reported [19]. In higher doses, in combination with midodrine and elderly patients, tolerance to medication is poor [20]. But in moderate doses, tolerance may be achieved [21].

Another potential medication is *Pyridostigmine*, a cholinesterase inhibitor that improves the sympathetic activity. It has less established results for the management of OH. Because of the modest effect, its use has been recommended in mild to moderate disease [22]. Starting dosage is 30 mg two to three times per day with titration up to 60 mg three times per day. The adverse effects include abdominal cramps, diarrhea, constipation, diaphoresis, sialorrhea, urinary incontinence, and fasciculations [23]. Pyridostigmine tolerance has not been studied in elderly patients in detail.

Atomoxetine is a noradrenaline reuptake inhibitor and is an emerging therapy for OH. It increases the noradrenaline concentration in the synaptic gap. The dosage is 18 mg/day for OH. Compared with midodrine, it produced a higher increase in upright systolic blood pressure in a randomized controlled trial [24]. Also, in neurogenic OH, it was demonstrated to be as effective as midodrine and better for ameliorating OH symptoms [25]. In elderly, the efficacy of atomoxetine in terms of ameliorating the orthostatic symptoms has not been evaluated in detail. Only in a previous case report, an improvement in blood pressure and symptoms over 10 weeks was presented [26]. In a recent study, the combination of atomoxetine and pyridostigmine has been effective in providing synergistic effects in increasing blood pressure in patients with autonomic failure that was unresponsive to separate medications. Also, this combination was associated with improvement in orthostatic symptoms and presented an alternative therapeutic option when there is no response to either drug alone [27]. The most common side effects are dry mouth, decreased appetite, nausea, and insomnia.

Yohimbine is an alpha-2 adrenergic antagonist, which increases sympathetic activity at the central nervous system. The available studies showed inconsistent results with this medication. The effect of yohimbine was compared with pyridostigmine on standing diastolic blood pressure and with a dosage of 5.4 mg/day. Yohimbine improved neurogenic OH-related symptoms [28]. But in another single-blind, crossover study with 17 patients, neither yohimbine nor atomoxetine alone increased blood pressure but coadministration of these two medications increased orthostatic tolerance [29]. No side effects have been reported with this medication, but the recommendation of yohimbine is low because of the inconsistent quality of evidence.

The other agents that have been tested for OH are *ergot alkaloids*, *fluoxetine*, *recombinant erythropoietin*, *ephedrine* and *ephedra alkaloids*, and *octreotide*. *Ergotamine* and its derivate dihydroergotamine increase blood pressure via alpha-adrenergic vasoconstriction of arteries and veins. Small-sized studies showed an increase for seated and upright blood pressure but because of limited data the recommendation for ergot alkaloids for treatment of OH is weak [30]. *Fluoxetine*, a selective serotonin reuptake inhibitor was evaluated in patients with neurogenic OH and Parkinson's disease and provided symptomatic relief [31]. Fluoxetine treatment for OH has a lower priority. *Recombinant erythropoietin* stimulates red cell mass production and increases circulating blood volume and tissue oxygenation. Especially in case of anemia, erythropoietin was evaluated for the treatment of OH, but for this medication, there is no randomized controlled trial. In the small-sized, open-label studies and case reports, its beneficial effect was observed [32]. But because of adverse events like allergic reactions, hypertension, and increased risk of thrombosis, the recommendation is poor.

Ephedrine is a nonspecific direct and indirect alpha- and beta-adrenoceptor agonist. It has been compared with midodrine. Although both midodrine and ephedrine increased supine systolic and diastolic blood pressures over placebo, the efficacy of midodrine was observed better than ephedrine [33]. Other ephedra alkaloids *Phenylpropanolamine* was investigated in an open-label study with pseudoephedrine. It significantly increased blood pressure in 13 patients [34]. Cerebral and cardiovascular events are the major safety problems, and the quality of evidence is weak. Subcutaneous administration of *Octreotide* somatostatin analog (12.5–25 µg/day) was investigated in the treatment of especially postprandial OH. The data for the administration of this medication on a regular basis is limited, but still, prevention of postprandial OH was replicated in further interventional studies with open-label design [35]. An improvement of OH in pre- and postexercise was observed also [35]. The quality of evidence for octreotide for neurogenic OH is very low but for postprandial OH is moderate. Because of adverse events, its use is not recommended in patients with diabetes mellitus [36–38].

For the control of postprandial OH, alpha-glycosidase inhibitors *acarbose* and *voglibose* were studied. In patients with type 2 diabetes mellitus and Parkinson's disease, acarbose significantly improved postprandial systolic blood pressure fall compared to placebo. Also, voglibose inhibited postprandial OH in a pre-post design study along with Parkinson's disease, diabetes mellitus, and elderly patients [39]. Hypoglycemia was not reported in patients with or without diabetes mellitus but most frequent adverse events were gastrointestinal symptoms. Although the recommendation is weak for voglibose, acarbose is strongly recommended for postprandial OH in patients with autonomic failure.

Caffeine was also evaluated in small patient groups, and it showed a favorable effect [40]. But based on available literature, the quality of evidence for caffeine to treat postprandial OH is very low. The following compounds, *indomethacin, ibuprofen*, and *methylphenidate* were evaluated for the treatment of OH, but evidence for the use of these compounds is quite weak. The favorable or unfavorable effects of all of these drugs were not studied in elderly patients.

Patients refractory to single medication may benefit from combination therapies. These combinations include midodrine plus fludrocortisone, ergotamine plus caffeine, midodrine or pseudoephedrine plus water bolus, and atomoxetine plus yohimbine [3].

When we review all of the non-pharmacological and pharmacological treatment modalities—regardless of patients' age—according to quality of evidence, the recommendations are as follows; In non-pharmacological interventions, abdominal and lower extremity compression binders have a moderate quality of evidence but are strongly recommended. Increasing sodium intake has low quality, but all other interventions also have a very low quality of evidence. Among pharmacological interventions, midodrine and droxidopa are strongly recommended, along with the high quality of evidence for midodrine and moderate quality of evidence for droxidopa. Atomoxetine and octreotide have a low quality of evidence and hence recommendations for them are weak. There is no significant quality of evidence for all other medications. Finally, acarbose and octreotide have strongly been recommended for postprandial hypotension [41]. In the elderly, these treatment modalities must be selected according to the priorities and benefits of each patient. But another important issue for elderly management is concomitant supine hypertension. As these events represent hemodynamic opposite medications that improve one condition may exacerbate the other. All management should be organized according to each patient's comorbidities, overall health status, and life expectancy. Advices are as follows: elevating the head of the bed and avoiding supine posture during the daytime if possible. Short-acting antihypertensive agents like captopril, losartan, clonidine, hydralazine, and nitroglycerin patch may be advised in patients with severe supine hypertension (up to 180/110 mmHg). Finally, for this group of patients, benefits and risks from every intervention should be evaluated and treatment should be individualized [4].

In conclusion, OH is a cardiovascular disorder evolving with autonomic nervous system dysfunction. Causes and possible numerous conditions have been identified on the patient basis. The studies predict risk factors and associated problems that are related to impaired prognosis. There is no good quality, randomized, placebo-controlled trial to provide proper guidance. The mainstay of management includes individually based non-pharmacological and pharmacological measures.

References

1. Magkas N, Tsioufis C, Thomopoulos C, et al. Orthostatic hypotension: from pathophysiology to clinical applications and therapeutic considerations. Clin Hypertens. 2019;21:546–54.
2. Wojszel ZB, Kasiukiewicz A, Magnuszewski L. Health and functional determinants of orthostatic hypotension in geriatric ward patients: a retrospective cross-sectional cohort study. J Nutr Health Aging. 2019;23:509–17.
3. Arnold AC, Raj SR. Orthostatic hypotension: a practical approach to investigation and management. Can J Cardiol. 2017;33:1725–8.
4. Gibbons CH, Schmidt P, Biaggioni I, et al. The recommendations of a consensus panel for the screening, diagnosis, and treatment of neurogenic orthostatic hypotension and associated supine hypertension. J Neurol. 2017;264:1567–82.
5. PRINT Research Group, Wright JT Jr, Williamson JD, et al. A randomized trial of intensive versus standard blood-pressure control. N Engl J Med. 2015;373:2103–16.
6. Gangavati A, Hajjar I, Quach L, et al. Hypertension, orthostatic hypotension, and the risk of falls in a community-dwelling elderly population: the maintenance of balance, independent living, intellect, and zest in the elderly of Boston study. J Am Geriatr Soc. 2011;59:383–9.
7. Brignole M, Moya A, de Lange FJ, et al. ESC Guidelines for the diagnosis and management of syncope. Eur Heart J. 2018;39:1883–948.
8. Juan J, Figueroa MD, Jeffrey R, Basford MD, Phillip A. Preventing and treating orthostatic hypotension: as easy as A, B, C. Cleve Clin J Med. 2010;77:298–306.
9. Rowell LB, Detry JM, Blackmon JR, Wyss C. Importance of the splanchnic vascular bed in human blood pressure regulation. J Appl Physiol. 1972;32:213–20.
10. Low PA, Singer W. Management of neurogenic orthostatic hypotension: an update. Lancet Neurol. 2008;7:451–8.
11. MacLean AR, Allen EV. Orthostatic hypotension and orthostatic tachycardia: treatment with the "head-up" bed. JAMA. 1940;115:2162–7.
12. Bonnin P, Ben Driss A, Benessiano J, et al. Enhanced flow-dependent vasodilatation after bed rest, a possible mechanism for orthostatic intolerance in humans. Eur J Appl Physiol. 2001;85:420–6.
13. Hale GM, Valdes J, Brenner M. The treatment of primary orthostatic hypotension. Ann Pharmacother. 2017;51:417–28.
14. Low PA, Gilden JL, Freeman R, et al. Efficacy of midodrine vs placebo in neurogenic orthostatic hypotension. A randomized, double-blind multicenter study. Midodrine Study Group. JAMA. 1997;277:1046–51.
15. Parsaik AK, Singh B, Altayar O, et al. Midodrine for orthostatic hypotension: a systematic review and meta-analysis of clinical trials. J Gen Intern Med. 2013;28:1496–503.
16. Gibbons CH, Schmidt P, Biaggioni I, et al. The recommendations of consensus panel for the screening, diagnosis, and treatment of neurogenic orthostatic hypotension and associated supine hypertension. J Neurol. 2017;264:567–82.
17. Hauser RA, Heritier S, Rowse GJ, et al. Droxidopa and reduced falls in a trial of Parkinson disease patients with neurogenic orthostatic hypotension. Clin Neuropharmacol. 2016;39:220–6.
18. Shen WK, Sheldon RS, Benditt DG, et al. ACC/AHA/HRS guideline for the evaluation and management of patients with syncope: a report of the American College of Cardiology/ American Heart Association Task Force on Clinical Practice Guidelines and the Heart Rhythm Society. Circulation. 2017;136:e60–e122.
19. Grijalva CG, Biaggioni I, Griffin MR, Shibao CA. Fludrocortisone is associated with a higher risk of all-cause hospitalizations compared with midodrine in patients with orthostatic hypotension. J Am Heart Assoc. 2017;6:e006848.
20. Hussain RM, McIntosh SJ, Lawson J, Kenny RA. Fludrocortisone in the treatment of hypotensive disorders in the elderly. Heart. 1996;76:507–9.
21. O'Brien H, Anne Kenny R. Syncope in the elderly. Eur Cardiol. 2014;9:28–36.

22. Singer W, Sandroni P, Opfer-Gehrking TL, et al. Pyridostigmine treatment trial in neurogenic orthostatic hypotension. Arch Neurol. 2006;63:513–8.
23. Bradley WG. Neurology in clinical practice. 5th ed. Philadelphia, PA: Butterworth-Heinemann/Elsevier; 2008.
24. Ramirez CE, Okamoto LE, Arnold AC, et al. Efficacy of atomoxetine versus midodrine for the treatment of orthostatic hypotension in autonomic failure. Hypertension. 2014;64:1235–40.
25. Byun JI, Kim DY, Moon J, et al. Efficacy of atomoxetine versus midodrine for neurogenic orthostatic hypotension. Ann Clin Transl Neurol. 2020;7:112–20.
26. Hale GM, Brenner M. Atomoxetine for orthostatic hypotension in an elderly patient over 10 weeks: a case report. Pharmacotherapy. 2015;35:e141–8.
27. Okamoto LE, Shibao CA, Gamboa A, et al. Synergistic pressor effect of atomoxetine and pyridostigmine in patients with neurogenic orthostatic hypotension. Hypertension. 2019;73:235–41.
28. Shibao C, Okamoto L, Gamboa A, et al. Comparative efficacy of yohimbine against pyridostigmine for the treatment of orthostatic hypotension in autonomic failure. Hypertension. 2010;56:847–51.
29. Okamoto L, Shibao C, Gamboa A, et al. Synergistic effect of norepinephrine transporter blockade and alpha-2 antagonism on blood pressure in autonomic failure. Hypertension. 2012;59:650–6.
30. Victor R, Talman W. Comparative effects of clonidine and dihydroergotamine on venomotor tone and orthostatic tolerance in patients with severe hypoadrenergic orthostatic hypotension. Am J Med. 2002;112:361–8.
31. Montastruc J, Pelat M, Verwaerde P, et al. Fluoxetine in orthostatic hypotension of Parkinson's disease: a clinical and experimental pilot study. Fundam Clin Pharmacol. 1998;12:398–402.
32. Kawakami K, Abe H, Harayama N, Nakashima Y. Successful treatment of severe orthostatic hypotension with erythropoietin. Pacing Clin Electrophysiol. 2003;26:105–7.
33. Fouad-Tarazi FM, Okabe M, Goren H. Alpha sympathomimetic treatment of autonomic insufficiency with orthostatic hypotension. Am J Med. 1995;99:604–10.
34. Jordan J, Shannon J, Diedrich A, et al. Water potentiates the pressor effect of ephedra alkaloids. Circulation. 2004;109:1823–5.
35. Smith G, Alam M, Watson L, Mathias C. Effect of the somatostatin analogue, octreotide, on exercise-induced hypotension in human subjects with chronic sympathetic failure. Clin Sci. 1995;89:367–73.
36. Mathias C, Fosbraey P, da Costa D, et al. The effect of desmopressin on nocturnal polyuria, overnight weight loss, and morning postural hypotension in patients with autonomic failure. Br Med J. 1986;293:353–4.
37. Sakakibara R, Matsuda S, Uchiyama T, et al. The effect of intranasal desmopressin on nocturnal waking in urination in multiple system atrophy patients with nocturnal polyuria. Clin Auton Res. 2003;13:106–8.
38. Alam M, Smith G, Bleasdale-Barr K, Pavitt DV, Mathias CJ. Effects of the peptide release inhibitor, octreotide, on daytime hypotension and on nocturnal hypertension in primary autonomic failure. J Hypertens. 1995;13:1664–9.
39. Maruta T, Komai K, Takamori M, Yamada M. Voglibose inhibits postprandial hypotension in neurologic disorders and elderly people. Neurology. 2006;66:1432–4.
40. Onrot J, Goldberg M, Biaggioni I, et al. Hemodynamic and humoral effects of caffeine in autonomic failure. Therapeutic implications for postprandial hypotension. N Engl J Med. 1985;313:549–55.
41. Eschlböck S, Wenning G, Fanciulli A. Evidence-based treatment of neurogenic orthostatic hypotension and related symptoms. Neural Transm. 2017;124:1567–605.

Orthostatic Hypertension

12

Suleyman Emre Kocyigit, Mehmet Selman Ontan, and Ahmet Turan Isik

Postural blood pressure changes appear to be a significant cause of morbidity and mortality in older adults. When moving from a lying to a standing position, a temporary decrease of blood pressure resolves quickly and without symptoms by the autonomic nervous system [1]. In older adults, this autonomic nervous system being affected may lead to postural blood pressure changes. Orthostatic hypotension (OH) is a postural blood pressure change most commonly studied in older adults with known etiology and pathophysiology [2]. OH affects 30% of the community-dwelling older adults [3], and it is emphasized that it may also be associated with geriatric syndromes such as frailty and malnutrition [4, 5], whereas orthostatic hypertension (OHT) is not clear in elderly, even though it has been stated that it may lead to some negative results in a small amount of studies.

12.1 Definition

There are no known consensus criteria for the diagnosis of OHT, as in OH. In different studies, different patient groups and different diagnostic criteria were performed. OHT is frequently regarded as an increase of more than 20 mmHg in systolic blood pressure when moving from supine position to standing position [6]. However, in some studies, the blood pressure in the supine position is <140/90 mmHg, while it is >140/90 mmHg in the standing position, and any increase in blood

S. E. Kocyigit
Department of Geriatric Medicine, Tepecik Training and Research Hospital, Izmir, Turkey

M. S. Ontan
Department of Internal Medicine, Faculty of Medicine, Dokuz Eylul University, Izmir, Turkey

A. T. Isik (✉)
Department of Geriatric Medicine, Faculty of Medicine, Dokuz Eylul University, Izmir, Turkey

© Springer Nature Switzerland AG 2021
A. T. Isik, P. Soysal (eds.), *Orthostatic Hypotension in Older Adults*,
https://doi.org/10.1007/978-3-030-62493-4_12

pressure in this range or only diastolic blood pressure is <90 mmHg in the supine position and is >90 mmHg in the standing position are also expressed as OHT [7, 8].

In addition, increases of 5 or 10 mmHg in postural isolated systolic blood pressure are also defined as OHT in studies [9, 10]. In addition, Kario suggests that when the increase in systolic blood pressure is over than 20 mmHg, there is an OHT diagnosis and that when it is over than 10 mmHg, there is a possible diagnosis of OHT [11]. In the literature, there are "active standing test," "head-up tilt table test (HUT)," and "ambulatory blood pressure monitoring (APBM)" which are used for the diagnosis of OHT. However, the time between the supine position and the standing position for postural blood pressure change varies according to the studies [6]. Home measurement of the active standing test for the diagnosis of OHT may be appropriate to eliminate the effect of the white coat and false OHT diagnosis [6]. ABPM can provide additional advantages in detecting short-term blood pressure changes [11, 12]. However, evaluation for HUT and OHT may be a good alternative. In a study for OH, HUT has been shown to be more preferable than AST, and HUT can be valuable for OHT [13]. Indeed, HUT has been used in many OHT studies. OHT can be asymptomatic in the elderly as well as presented with orthostatism symptoms [6, 14]. Consensus criteria are required for the diagnostic criteria, for which the findings should be supported by randomized controlled studies.

12.2 Pathophysiology

The pathophysiology of OHT is not clearly understood. However, there are several possible mechanisms mentioned in the literature. It is thought that autonomic nerve dysfunction is in the foreground [15]. OHT may occur due to extreme sympathetic warning against gravity as a result of the change of position. As a result, intense peripheral vasoconstriction develops. In addition, a decrease in venous pooling and venous return occurring when standing up can also lead to a decrease in cardiac output, whereas an increase in sympathetic stimulation can also lead to OHT [6, 11]. Disruption in baroreceptor reflex sensitivity, essential hypertension, diabetes mellitus, neurological diseases, and arterial stiffness and RAAS activation as a result of aging, alpha-adrenergic vascular hyperactivity, and increased vasopressin secretion may also lead to sympathetic nerve stimulation and/or peripheral vasoconstriction [6, 11, 16]. As a result of a decrease in cardiac output, baroreceptor hypersensitivity develops, which may contribute to excessive sympathetic activation [6]. Kario and Shimada found that circulating levels of vasopressin in extreme dippers are higher following a head-up tilt challenge than in dippers and non-dippers, but extreme dippers did not have significantly higher levels of norepinephrine or plasma renin activity [17]. In some studies, the high rate of urinary norepinephrine levels in patients with OHT compared to those without OHT also supports increased sympathetic activity [18]. The factors that trigger the development of OHT are still unclear. Furthermore, OHT and postural tachycardia syndrome (POTS) can be seen together [6]. In a significant portion of cases with POTS, plasma norepinephrine levels that are high in a standing position show an extreme sympathetic response to orthostatic stress, which are defined as a hyperadrenergic type POTS [19, 20]. Patients with OHT may develop hyperadrenergic POTS. In addition, RAAS activation, pheochromocytoma, mast cell activation, and norepinephrine transport deficiency, which develop as a result of decreased kidney blood flow, can also lead to OHT [6].

12.3   Epidemiology and Clinical Significance

The prevalence of OHT varies considerably in the literature. The difference in the measurement method used, the changes in the diagnostic criteria, and the differences in the quality of the population studied affect changes in prevalence. In a study, the prevalence was determined as 16.2% [21], while the change in systolic blood pressure was taken as >20 mmHg, and the ratio varies between 1.1% and 28% [6]. There are also studies showing that the frequency of OHT increases significantly in individuals with diabetes and hypertension compared to nondiabetic and normotensive. Sympathetic abnormalities, peripheral vascular disease, baroreceptor failure, silent cerebral disease, and chronic kidney disease can also facilitate the development of OHT in the elderly [21].

It is also stated that OHT is associated with hypertensive target organ damage. In addition, while there is information in the literature that OHT may have an increased cardiovascular risk, there are studies showing that the left atrium volume is lower in OHT patients and there will be no harmful phenomenon [22]. It is also stated to be a risk factor for masked hypertension [23] that OHT may be more common in those with extreme dipper hypertension, which may be related to cerebrovascular damage [24]. In the literature, OHT has been shown to be predictive for cerebrovascular disease in older individuals [11]. It is pointed out that in hypertensives with OHT, silent lacunar infarction and deep white matter damage are higher than hypertensives without OHT [25]. There are contradictory studies showing the effect of OHT on mortality risk. In a study showing the effect of OHT on all-cause mortality in hospitalized elderly individuals by Weiss et al., it was shown that the survival was better in elderly people with OHT, and in another study, there was no increase in mortality in very elderly individuals, while Kostis et al. claim that mortality risk is higher in OHT cases compared to the control group, and cardiovascular risk may be reduced by early detection [26, 27]. There is also information that it is associated with urinary albumin excretion and high BNP [28]. In the elderly without diabetes, there was no significant difference between OHT and plasma fibrinogen and carotid intima-media thickness compared to the control group [29]. The case study is also reported in the literature that OHT may develop in combination with renal artery stenosis and nephroptosis [30]. Examining the cognitive effect of orthostatic blood pressure on the elderly, the Progetto Veneto Anziani study showed that OHT could predict cognitive decline but OH could not [31]. However, this idea was achieved only by changes in MMSE values, since there is no evidence that it shows the risk of dementia. These findings should be supported by further studies. In addition,

OHT was found to be associated with early stage neuropathy in normotensive diabetic patients [7]. Jannetta et al. highlighted that there is a relationship between hypertension, including orthostatic hypertension, and medullary vascular compression [32].

12.4   Management and Treatment

There is no specific and accepted treatment for OHT. However, considering the literature, it can be thought that certain treatment methods can be effective. Primarily, non-pharmacological approaches as in OH may be beneficial in patients presenting with orthostatism symptoms. For example, when considering that venous pooling is involved in pathophysiology, compression stockings may be useful to reduce the pooling. Correction of the underlying conditions can also treat OHT [6]. For example, if there is masked hypertension or essential hypertension on the ground, effective blood pressure regulation may regress OHT, or if diabetes mellitus is present—there are publications indicating that OHT is common in these patients—blood sugar regulation can improve OHT [6]. Therefore, in cases where OHT is detected, evaluation of blood pressure and blood sugar becomes important. Renal vascularization may be brought up if renal artery stenosis is accompanied. Patients with OHT should be carefully evaluated in terms of cerebrovascular events, and appropriate diagnostic methods should be used in skeptical cases.

In the study showing the effect of doxazosin, which is an alpha-blocker, on OHT, it has been shown that it can control OHT and protect it from target organ damage as a result of adding 1 mg of doxazosin and applying it up to 4 mg dose with monthly intervals until the blood pressure target is <130/85 mmHg [28, 33].

In small case series, clonidine has been shown to be beneficial in patients with symptomatic OHT with baroreflex deficiency due to its sympatholytic properties [34]. In a large observational study, systolic and diastolic blood pressures were slightly reduced, while pulse pressures remained unchanged due to a standing pressure effect of beta-blockers. However, their effects remain uncertain as they can worsen OHT [35]. Thoracic sympathectomy has also been demonstrated to correct OHT in small case series, but it should be kept in mind that there will be a risk of OH [36]. Transdermal nitroglycerin administered at bedtime reduces supine BP substantially in patients with autonomic failure. Therefore, it may be useful for OHT, but further studies are needed on this topic [37]. It has been shown that OHT is eliminated by surgical intervention in cases with OHT due to nephroptosis, but it is not routinely used because it is a high-risk operation [30]. Finally, it seems more rational to take the necessary precautions in the symptomatic state of OHT, whose treatment modality is not clear, and to combat comorbid diseases.

12.5   Conclusion

Randomized controlled studies with high sample size are not required to demonstrate the effect of OHT, whose diagnostic criteria, clinical significance, and treatment are not clear on the geriatric population. There are various clues about the effect of OHT in the literature, and broader and different findings need to be revealed.

References

1. Ricci F, De Caterina R, Fedorowski A. Orthostatic hypotension: epidemiology, prognosis, and treatment. J Am Coll Cardiol. 2015;66(7):848–60.
2. Kanjwal K, George A, Figueredo VM, Grubb BP. Orthostatic hypotension: definition, diagnosis and management. J Cardiovasc Med (Hagerstown). 2015;16(2):75–81. https://doi.org/10.2459/01.JCM.0000446386.01100.35.
3. Frith J, Parry SW. New horizons in orthostatic hypotension. Age Ageing. 2017;46(2):168–74. https://doi.org/10.1093/ageing/afw211.
4. Kocyigit SE, Soysal P, Bulut EA, Aydin AE, Dokuzlar O, Isik AT. What is the relationship between frailty and orthostatic hypotension in older adults? J Geriatr Cardiol. 2019;16(3):272–9. https://doi.org/10.11909/j.issn.1671-5411.2019.03.005.
5. Kocyigit SE, Soysal P, Ates Bulut E, Isik AT. Malnutrition and malnutrition risk can be associated with systolic orthostatic hypotension in older adults. J Nutr Health Aging. 2018;22(8):928–33. https://doi.org/10.1007/s12603-018-1032-6.
6. Magkas N, Tsioufis C, Thomopoulos C, Dilaveris P, Georgiopoulos G, Doumas M, Papadopoulos D, Tousoulis D. Orthostatic hypertension: from pathophysiology to clinical applications and therapeutic considerations. J Clin Hypertens. 2019;21(3):426–33. https://doi.org/10.1111/jch.13491.
7. Yoshinari M, Wakisaka M, Nakamura U, Yoshioka M, Uchizono Y, Iwase M. Orthostatic hypertension in patients with type 2 diabetes. Diabetes Care. 2001;24(10):1783–6.
8. Streeten DH, Auchincloss JH Jr, Anderson GH Jr, Richardson RL, Thomas FD, Miller JW. Orthostatic hypertension. Pathogenetic studies. Hypertension. 1985;7(2):196–203.
9. Tabara Y, Igase M, Miki T, Ohyagi Y, Matsuda F, Kohara K, J-SHIPP Study Group. Orthostatic hypertension as a predisposing factor for masked hypertension: the J-SHIPP study. Hypertens Res. 2016;39(9):664–9. https://doi.org/10.1038/hr.2016.43.
10. Thomas RJ, Liu K, Jacobs DR Jr, Bild DE, Kiefe CI, Hulley SB. Positional change in blood pressure and 8-year risk of hypertension: the CARDIA study. Mayo Clin Proc. 2003;78(8):951–8.
11. Kario K. Orthostatic hypertension – a new haemodynamic cardiovascular risk factor. Nat Rev Nephrol. 2013;9(12):726–38.
12. Brignole M, Moya A, de Lange FJ, et al. 2018 ESC Guidelines for the diagnosis and management of syncope. Eur Heart J. 2018;39(21):1883–948.
13. Aydin AE, Soysal P, Isik AT. Which is preferable for orthostatic hypotension diagnosis in older adults: active standing test or head-up tilt table test? Clin Interv Aging. 2017;12:207–12. https://doi.org/10.2147/CIA.S129868.
14. Lee H, Kim HA. Orthostatic hypertension: an underestimated cause of orthostatic intolerance. Clin Neurophysiol. 2016;127(4):2102–7.
15. Robertson D. Orthostatic hypertension: the last hemodynamic frontier. Hypertension. 2011;57(2):158–9.
16. Fessel J, Robertson D. Orthostatic hypertension: when pressor reflexes overcompensate. Nat Clin Pract Nephrol. 2006;2(8):424–31.

17. Kario K, Shimada K. Risers and extreme-dippers of nocturnal blood pressure in hypertension: antihypertensive strategy for nocturnal blood pressure. Clin Exp Hypertens. 2004;26(2):177–89.
18. Vriz O, Soon G, Lu H, Weder AB, Canali C, Palatini P. Does ortho-static testing have any role in the evaluation of the young subject with mild hypertension?: an insight from the HARVEST study. Am J Hypertens. 1997;10(5 Pt 1):546–51.
19. Benarroch EE. Postural tachycardia syndrome: a heterogeneous and multifactorial disorder. Mayo Clin Proc. 2012;87(12):1214–25.
20. Low PA, Sandroni P, Joyner M, Shen WK. Postural tachycardia syndrome (POTS). J Cardiovasc Electrophysiol. 2009;20(3):352–8.
21. Mesquita P, Queiroz D, Lamartine de Lima Silva V, Texeira Vde C, Vilaça de Lima YR, Júnior ER, Garcia J, Bandeira F. Prevalence of orthostatic hypertension in elderly patients with type 2 diabetes. Int J Endocrinol. 2015;2015:463487. https://doi.org/10.1155/2015/463487.
22. Buddineni JP, Chauhan L, Ahsan ST, Whaley-Connell A. An emerging role for understanding orthostatic hypertension in the cardiorenal syndrome. Cardiorenal Med. 2011;1(2):113–22. https://doi.org/10.1159/000327141.
23. Barochiner J, Cuffaro PE, Aparicio LS, et al. Predictors of masked hypertension among treated hypertensive patients: an interesting association with orthostatic hypertension. Am J Hypertens. 2013;26(7):872–8.
24. Kario K, Eguchi K, Nakagawa Y, Motai K, Shimada K. Relationship between extreme dippers and orthostatic hypertension in elderly hypertensive patients. Hypertension. 1998;31(1):77–82.
25. Kario K, Eguchi K, Hoshide S, Hoshide Y, Umeda Y, Mitsuhashi T, Shimada K. U-curve relationship between orthostatic blood pressure change and silent cerebrovascular disease in elderly hypertensives: orthostatic hypertension as a new cardiovascular risk factor. J Am Coll Cardiol. 2002;40(1):133–41.
26. Weiss A, Beloosesky Y, Grossman A, Shlesinger A, Koren-Morag N, Grossman E. The association between orthostatic hypertension and all- cause mortality in hospitalized elderly persons. J Geriatr Cardiol. 2016;13(3):239–43. https://doi.org/10.11909/j.issn.1671-5411.2016.03.004.
27. Kostis WJ, Sargsyan D, Mekkaoui C, Moreyra AE, Cabrera J, Cosgrove NM, Sedjro JE, Kostis JB, Cushman WC, Pantazopoulos JS, Pressel SL, Davis BR. Association of orthostatic hypertension with mortality in the Systolic Hypertension in the Elderly Program. J Hum Hypertens. 2019;33(10):735–40. https://doi.org/10.1038/s41371-019-0180-4.
28. Kario K, Matsui Y, Shibasaki S, Eguchi K, Ishikawa J, Hoshide S, Ishikawa S, Kabutoya T, Schwartz JE, Pickering TG, Shimada K, Japan Morning Surge-1 (JMS-1) Study Group. An alpha-adrenergic blocker titrated by self-measured blood pressure recordings lowered blood pressure and microalbuminuria in patients with morning hypertension: the Japan Morning Surge-1 Study. J Hypertens. 2008;26(6):1257–65. https://doi.org/10.1097/HJH.0b013e3282fd173c.
29. Fedorowski A, Ostling G, Persson M, Struck J, Engström G, Nilsson PM, Hedblad B, Melander O. Orthostatic blood pressure response, carotid intima-media thickness, and plasma fibrinogen in older nondiabetic adults. J Hypertens. 2012;30(3):522–9. https://doi.org/10.1097/HJH.0b013e32834fa860.
30. Tsukamoto Y, Komuro Y, Akutsu F, et al. Orthostatic hypertension due to coexistence of renal fibromuscular dysplasia and nephroptosis. Jpn Circ J. 1988;52(12):1408–14.
31. Curreri C, Giantin V, Veronese N, Trevisan C, Sartori L, Musacchio E, Zambon S, Maggi S, Perissinotto E, Corti MC, Crepaldi G, Manzato E, Sergi G. Orthostatic changes in blood pressure and cognitive status in the elderly: the Progetto Veneto Anziani study. Hypertension. 2016;68(2):427–35. https://doi.org/10.1161/HYPERTENSIONAHA.
32. Jannetta PJ, Segal R, Wolfson SK Jr. Neurogenic hypertension: etiology and surgical treatment. I. Observations in 53 patients. Ann Surg. 1985;201(3):391–8.
33. Hoshide S, Parati G, Matsui Y, Shibazaki S, Eguchi K, Kario K. Orthostatic hypertension: home blood pressure monitoring for detection and assessment of treatment with doxazosin. Hypertens Res. 2012;35(1):100–6.
34. Robertson D, Hollister AS, Biaggioni I, Netterville JL, Mosqueda-Garcia R, Robertson RM. The diagnosis and treatment of baroreflex failure. N Engl J Med. 1993;329(20):1449–55.

35. Cleophas TJ, Grabowsky I, Niemeyer MG, Mäkel WM, van der Wall EE, Nebivolol Follow-Up Study Group. Paradoxical pressor effects of beta-blockers in standing elderly patients with mild hypertension: a beneficial side effect. Circulation. 2002;105(14):1669–71.
36. Suzuki T, Masuda Y, Nonaka M, Kadokura M, Hosoyamada A. Endoscopic thoracic sympathectomy attenuates reflex tachycardia during head-up tilt in lightly anesthetized patients with essential plamar hyperhidrosis. J Anesth. 2002;16(1):4–8.
37. Jordan J, Shannon JR, Pohar B, Paranjape SY, Robertson D, Robertson RM, Biaggioni I. Contrasting effects of vasodilators on blood pressure and sodium balance in the hypertension of autonomic failure. J Am Soc Nephrol. 1999;10(1):35–42.

Other Syndromes of Orthostatic Intolerance: Delayed Orthostatic Hypotension, Postprandial Hypotension, Postural Orthostatic Tachycardia Syndrome, and Reflex Syncope

13

Artur Fedorowski, Viktor Hamrefors, and Fabrizio Ricci

13.1 Delayed and Postprandial Orthostatic Hypotension

Beyond classical orthostatic hypotension (OH), the gravitational force may contribute to other forms of orthostatic intolerance and delayed and postprandial OH. In delayed OH, the significant blood pressure (BP) drop occurs first after 3-min period of orthostasis, whereas in postprandial OH, the symptoms appear first approximately 15–30 min after the meal. These two special forms of orthostatic intolerance are frequently identified in older individuals with unexplained syncope and negative initial workup including active standing test and ECG monitoring. Usually, more advanced tests have to be performed, such as head-up tilt testing (HUT) with beat-to-beat BP monitoring and 24-h ambulatory BP monitoring (ABPM) with detailed analysis of individual data, especially in the postprandial period.

A. Fedorowski (✉)
Department of Cardiology, Skåne University Hospital, Malmö, Sweden

Department of Clinical Sciences, Lund University, Malmö, Sweden
e-mail: artur.fedorowski@med.lu.se

V. Hamrefors
Department of Clinical Sciences, Lund University, Malmö, Sweden

Department of Internal Medicine, Skåne University Hospital, Malmö, Sweden
e-mail: viktor.hamrefors@med.lu.se

F. Ricci
Department of Clinical Sciences, Lund University, Malmö, Sweden

Department of Neuroscience, Imaging and Clinical Sciences, "G. d'Annunzio" University, Chieti, Italy
e-mail: fabrizio.ricci@unich.it

© Springer Nature Switzerland AG 2021
A. T. Isik, P. Soysal (eds.), *Orthostatic Hypotension in Older Adults*,
https://doi.org/10.1007/978-3-030-62493-4_13

13.1.1 Delayed Orthostatic Hypotension

Delayed orthostatic hypotension is defined as a slow progressive drop in BP $\geq20/10$ mmHg (or $\geq30/15$ mmHg in patients with arterial hypertension) occurring first after 3 min of active standing or, for the most accurate diagnosis, after 3 min of HUT [1, 2]. This condition has been associated with milder abnormalities of sympathetic adrenergic function, suggesting that this disorder may be a less severe or an early form of autonomic failure, along with age-related impairment of compensatory reflexes and with a stiffer, more preload-dependent heart in older patients [2, 3]. The absence of bradycardia or pauses usually differentiates delayed OH from reflex syncope, although mixed forms are often encountered in clinical practice [4].

13.1.1.1 Prevalence and Clinical Significance of Delayed OH

Delayed OH was first described by Streeten and Anderson [5], but there is limited data on pathophysiology and differences between classical and delayed OH. Current evidence supports the perspective of delayed OH as an early and milder phenotype of autonomic dysfunction preceding classical OH and presenting at younger age with less severe abnormalities of both autonomic and neuroendocrine control mechanisms [3, 6]. On a pathophysiological basis, it seems likely that delayed OH is a consequence of increased peripheral venous pooling, increased fluid transudation, along with gradual failure of sympathetic adrenergic system and humoral mechanisms that counteract the redistribution of blood volume [6].

Similar to classical OH, delayed OH can be classified into two broad categories dealing with structural (neurogenic) or functional (non-neurogenic) causes of autonomic nervous system failure [2]. Neurogenic etiologies include Parkinson's disease, α-synucleinopathies, and other primary neurodegenerative disorders and can also be seen in autonomic nervous system failure secondary to diabetes, amyloidosis, renal failure, or in autoimmune diseases.

Factors that may cause functional impairment of the autonomic nervous system include aging, treatment with diuretics, tricyclic antidepressants or chemotherapeutic agents, absolute or relative reduction of circulating blood volume, venous pooling, and use of inotropic and/or chronotropic heart failure medications. Delayed OH has been also reported to occur after surgical denervation of the carotid sinus baroreceptors and with drugs interfering with vasoconstrictor mechanisms, such as central sympathetic outflow blocking agents and α-blockers, indicating that impaired baroreflex function is commonly implicated [7]. Overall, only a minority of patients with delayed OH demonstrate clinically overt neurogenic disease, and at least 40% cases of moderate or severe OH are eventually classified as idiopathic.

While both forms of classical and delayed OH are generally considered as a common finding in older populations, estimates of their prevalence can vary widely. In a pooled analysis of observational studies, it has been shown that OH affects nearly one in five older community-dwelling individuals and almost one in four persons living in long-term residential care facilities [8]. However, despite the availability of consensus guidelines, there is still large inter-study heterogeneity in assessment methods used to measure orthostatic BP, where continuous versus intermittent monitoring and the lack of a clear definition for what constitutes a sustained drop in BP make it difficult to get reliable estimates of disease prevalence.

In a cohort of 230 consecutive symptomatic patients undergoing 60° head-up tilt for 45 min, of 108 patients with OH, only 46% had OH within 3 min, while delayed OH occurred in 54% of the tested population and was associated with milder abnormalities of sympathetic adrenergic function [6]. Particularly, patients with delayed OH beyond 10 min were younger and presented with smaller BP falls during phase II of the Valsalva maneuver and greater phase IV overshoot, suggesting a milder or early phenotype of sympathetic adrenergic failure [6]. Long-term follow-up of the same cohort revealed that over 10 years, more than half of subjects with delayed OH developed classical OH phenotype and a sizeable proportion received a neurodegenerative disease diagnosis. Of note, as delayed OH frequently progresses to OH and combines with diabetes, abnormal autonomic tests, or overt α-synucleinopathies, it heralds higher all-cause mortality [9]. Despite the fact that mortality is associated with the development of specific underlying diseases, progression to OH magnifies the risk, particularly in individuals with diabetes, in whom delayed OH entails fourfold higher mortality than diabetes alone [9]. Delayed OH falls along the continuum of morbidity and mortality associated with CV autonomic dysfunction. The concept of CV disease continuum framed as a chain of events, initiated by a number of risk factors and progressing through different physiologic pathways up to the development of end-stage heart disease, has been proposed and validated through the evidence that an intervention at any point along this chain can modify the course of the disease also providing cardioprotective effects [10].

It is now increasingly recognized that a direct relationship exists between OH and each step of the cascade of pathophysiologic and clinical events in the CV disease continuum [11].

13.1.1.2   Diagnosis

Changing from the supine to the upright position produces a displacement of blood from the thorax to the lower limbs and abdominal cavity that leads to a decrease in venous return and cardiac output. In the absence of compensatory mechanisms, a fall in BP may lead to syncope. According to the consensus statement, endorsed by the American Autonomic Society, the European Federation of Autonomic Societies, the Autonomic Research Group of the World Federation of Neurology, the Autonomic Disorders section of the American Academy of Neurology [1], and the European Society of Cardiology [12], delayed OH may be revealed in patients with suspected orthostatic hypotension by extending the period of orthostatic stress (active standing or HUT) beyond 3 min.

Hypo-responsiveness of cardiovascular (CV) autonomic regulatory systems underlying delayed OH is relatively easy to detect by applying noninvasive beat-to-beat BP measurement and Valsalva maneuver [13]. According to the standard examination protocol, patients take their regular medications and fast for ≥2 h before the test, but they are allowed to drink water. The examination includes basic CV autonomic testing (typically Valsalva maneuver and active standing) and HUT according to the Italian protocol i.e., a drug-free HUT phase of 20 min or until syncope occurred, under continuous ECG and beat-to-beat BP monitoring. If the drug-free phase is negative, 400 μg sublingual nitroglycerin is administered and the patient is monitored for another 15 min. This part of the protocol is usually reserved for patients with unexplained syncope, in whom the passive phase is inconclusive and standing systolic BP (SBP) is still above 90 mmHg. However, the hemodynamic response during the drug-potentiated HUT phase is not a part of OH evaluation. While classical OH is defined as a sustained decrease in SBP ≥20 mmHg or diastolic BP (DBP) ≥10 mmHg during first 3 min of HUT, presence of delayed OH assumes that significant BP fall occurs first after 3 min of HUT (Fig. 13.1), excluding the obvious pattern of vasovagal reflex presenting with a typical prodrome and bradycardia preceding or coinciding with a significant BP fall. A pathologic Valsalva maneuver is defined based on the absence of an increase in heart rate during phase II, absence of late phase II BP recovery, and delayed BP recovery without the characteristic overshoot during phase IV [3]. Pathologic Valsalva test pattern implies presence of structural damage to the efferent arm of sympathetic system.

While the prognostic value of 24-h ambulatory blood pressure monitoring (ABPM) in arterial hypertension is fully established, the applicability of ABPM in CV autonomic dysfunction remains limited, and validated criteria for the ambulatory screening of OH with ABPM are yet to be determined. However, ABPM might provide additional insights into BP alterations associated with OH, including

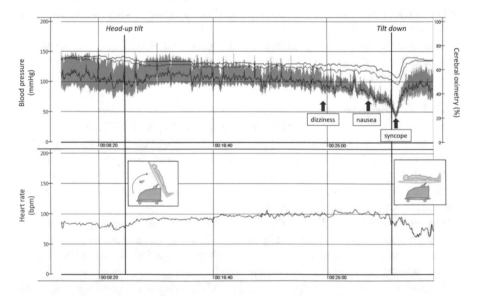

Fig. 13.1 Delayed orthostatic hypotension. Beat-to-beat blood pressure (mmHg) and cerebral oxygen saturation (%) in the upper panel with heart rate (bpm) depicted in red in the lower panel during head-up tilt in a representative patient (man, 80-year old) with delayed orthostatic hypotension leading to an onset of vasovagal reflex and syncope. (Modified from: Torabi P, Ricci F, Hamrefors V, Sutton R, Fedorowski A. Classical and Delayed Orthostatic Hypotension in Patients With Unexplained Syncope and Severe Orthostatic Intolerance. Front Cardiovasc Med 2020;7:21)

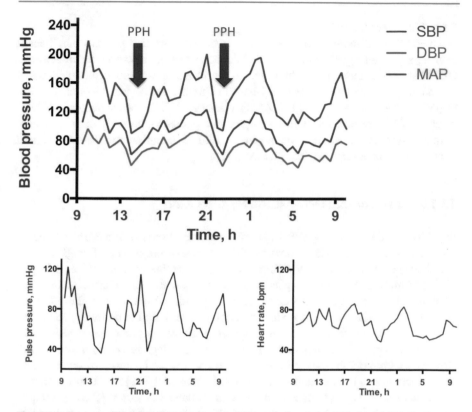

Fig. 13.2 Postprandial orthostatic hypotension. Twenty-four-hour ambulatory blood pressure monitoring documenting two symptomatic postprandial hypotension episodes in an 88-year-old woman with hypertension and history of syncope. *DBP* diastolic blood pressure, *MAP* mean arterial blood pressure, *PPH* postprandial hypotension, *SBP* systolic blood pressure

awakening hypotension, postprandial hypotension (Fig. 13.2), nocturnal reverse dipping, and nocturnal hypertension [14]. Particularly, high nocturnal BP values and 24-h weighted BP variability have been associated with OH, and two specific parameters for the ambulatory screening of OH with ABPM have been recently proposed, including [15]:

1. ≥2 hypotensive episodes, defined as an SBP drop ≥15 mmHg, compared to the average 24-h SBP and
2. presence of awakening hypotension, defined as an SBP drop ≥15 mmHg within 90 min after getting up in the morning compared to the average 24-h SBP.

Further tests, such as supine/standing catecholamines, imaging of the brain and of cardiac sympathetic nerves, may be indicated to confirm peripheral noradrenergic denervation or central neurodegenerative process, all of which are usually performed in specialized tertiary care units [16–18].

13.1.1.3 Treatment

Delayed OH is difficult to treat, and there is no evidence that patients may benefit from a particular drug class in terms of CV risk protection. However, as for classical OH, control of symptoms can be obtained by means of both non-pharmacological and pharmacological measures (see Chap. 11) greatly enhancing the quality of life of patients with delayed OH [19]. As for classical OH, the pharmacological treatment should be reserved to highly symptomatic patients with daily or at least very frequent symptoms, whereas management of less symptomatic patients should focus upon nonpharmacological measures [2].

13.1.2 Postprandial Orthostatic Hypotension

In postprandial hypotension (PPH), BP fall typically occurs within 2 h after a meal. Over the years, various definitions of PPH have been proposed, although none is based on normative data or CV risk estimates. Most authors define PPH as a drop in SBP $\geq$20 mmHg or alternatively as continuous SBP <90 mmHg, after having been >100 mmHg before the meal—either occurring within 2 h after completion of the meal. However, there is still a noticeable degree of variation in defining PPH [20].

PPH is more frequently observed in elderly patients with neurologic comorbidities, and as most of the patients are asymptomatic, the diagnosis is often overlooked. However, all physicians caring for elderly patients should be aware of the hypotensive effects of food intake and should carefully consider PPH in the evaluation of syncope, falls, and symptoms of orthostatic intolerance [21]. As a general principle, treatment should be geared to patients' symptoms and their impact on daily function rather than targeting a definite BP cutoff. Optimal treatment of symptomatic PPH includes the same principles reported for OH and should aim to correct precipitating factors, such as avoidance of volume depletion, and down-titration/withdrawal of offending medications that can cause or exacerbate OH, such as of diuretics, alpha-blockers, beta-blockers, selective serotonin reuptake inhibitors, antipsychotics, vasodilators, sedatives, hypnotics, phosphodiesterase, inhibitors, or muscle relaxant drugs [22]. Modification of meals (avoiding large and high-carbohydrate meals) and liberalization of salt and fluid intake may be helpful in selected patients [21, 23]. Particularly, PPH can be minimized by avoiding large and high-carbohydrate meals, alcohol intake and activities or sudden standing immediately after eating. Conversely, generous intake of water with meals or rapid ingestion of cool water have been reported to be effective in treating orthostatic intolerance and PPH [24].

Should nonpharmacologic measures reveal insufficient to prevent symptoms, particularly in moderate/severe forms of disease, pharmacologic intervention, can be recommended. Of note, acarbose, an alpha-glucosidase inhibitor, and octreotide, a somatostatin analogue, were found to attenuate PPH in small trials of patients with autonomic failure [25, 26]. Nevertheless, beneficial effects of medications have been demonstrated for BP response, but not for symptomatic improvement [27].

13.2 Postural Orthostatic Tachycardia Syndrome

Postural orthostatic tachycardia syndrome (POTS) is a common variant of CV autonomic dysfunction diagnosed by a characteristic excessive heart rate increase on standing associated with symptoms of orthostatic intolerance and occasional syncope [1, 12, 28, 29]. The syndrome affects predominantly younger women (≈80–85%) [28, 30]. POTS is extremely rare in older population as the majority of patients report onset of disease before the age of 30 [31], although the symptoms may be persistent and span beyond the sixth decade of life. Usually, postural tachycardia is attenuated when the POTS patients get older as the maximal heart rate declines with advancing age, from 200 beats per minute (bpm) in the age of 20–160 bpm in the age of 60 [32]. The long-term prospective studies of POTS are not available.

The term POTS was coined in 1993 by a team from Mayo Clinic (Rochester, MN, USA) to illustrate a phenomenon of sudden-onset pandysautonomia with prevailing hyperadrenergic circulatory symptoms and abnormal orthostatic heart rate acceleration [33]. The Mayo Clinic group proposed diagnostic criteria of POTS: heart rate increase >30 bpm or above 120 bpm within first 5 min after assuming standing position, accompanied by symptoms of orthostatic intolerance [34]. These criteria were subsequently adopted with some modifications by major neurologic, autonomic, and cardiologic societies [1, 12, 28].

13.2.1 Diagnosis

The current diagnostic criteria for POTS are summarized in Table 13.1. To establish POTS diagnosis, one should perform repeated active standing tests after resting in supine position for at least 5 min, and record BP and heart rate after 1, 3, 5, and 10 min of standing. Tests performed after large meals, physical exercise, and coffee consumption should be avoided. POTS may overlap vasovagal syncope, panic disorders, psychogenic pseudosyncope, chronic fatigue syndrome, Ehlers-Danlos syndrome, and paroxysmal supraventricular arrhythmias, which should be kept in mind in complex cases [12, 28, 30, 35].

A typical patient with POTS is a young woman about 15–30 years old, although one-fifth are males [36, 37]. Notably, symptoms of orthostatic intolerance, palpitations, and number of syncopal events do not well discriminate POTS from OH and recurrent vasovagal syncope [37]. The onset of POTS may be precipitated by viral infection, vaccination, trauma, pregnancy, surgery, or even a period of intensive psychosocial stress [29, 38–41]. A substantial number of POTS patients do not recall any triggering event and experience rather slowly progressing or even stationary symptoms over a long period of time [36]. In patients diagnosed with joint hypermobility syndrome, a variant of Ehlers-Danlos syndrome, the onset of POTS may be rather insidious and the symptoms may develop over years beginning with teenage [42].

Table 13.1 Diagnostic criteria of postural orthostatic tachycardia syndrome

The diagnostic criteria	Endorsed by:
Sustained heart rate increment of not less than *30* bpm or above *120* bpm within 10 min of active standing or head-up tilt	American Academy of Neurology American Autonomic Society American College of Cardiology
Absence of OH (i.e., sustained SBP drop of not less than 20 mmHg)	American Heart Association European Federation of Autonomic Societies
Reproduction of spontaneous symptoms such as lightheadedness, palpitations, tremulousness, generalized weakness, blurred vision, and fatigue. In some patients, postural tachycardia may induce vasovagal syncope corresponding to spontaneous attacks from patient's history	European Heart Rhythm Association European Society of Cardiology Heart Rhythm Society
History of chronic orthostatic intolerance and other typical POTS-associated symptoms (for at least 6 months[a])	
Absence of other conditions associated with sinus tachycardia, such as anxiety disorders, hyperventilation, anemia, fever, pain, infection, dehydration, hyperthyroidism, pheochromocytoma, use of cardioactive drugs (sympathomimetics, anticholinergics)	

[a]Symptoms of shorter duration should be reevaluated to confirm the diagnosis

The predominant and pathognomonic feature of POTS is *chronic orthostatic intolerance*, usually exacerbated by high ambient temperature, morning hours, insufficient fluid intake, dehydration, physical strain, large meals, and occasional infection with fever. POTS patients typically present with a spectrum of symptoms which are detailed in Table 13.2. The broad-spectrum panorama in POTS and similarities with other less defined conditions such as chronic fatigue syndrome make the diagnosis difficult for an unexperienced doctor [29]. The most common complaints are dizziness while standing, body weakness, rapid heartbeat and palpitation on standing, headache, fatigue, abdominal pain, mental impairment, and syncope [35, 38, 43–46]. Syncope or transient loss of consciousness is very common in POTS, affecting approximately one-third of patients [47–50].

As mentioned above, the diagnosis of POTS is difficult as it usually requires both doctor's vigilance combined with knowledge about the syndrome and an access to CV autonomic tests. A complicating factor is heterogeneity of symptoms that may mask the underlying POTS and divert clinician's attention towards other conditions with a similar presentation such as anxiety disorders, hyperthyroidism, anemia, pheochromocytoma, asthenia, orthostatic hypotension, hypocortisolemia, and other endocrinological disorders. An active standing test may immediately give a diagnostic clue, if supported by a history of characteristic chronic orthostatic intolerance, postural heart rhythm acceleration, and varying panorama of accompanying complaints (Table 13.2). When the symptoms are more severe, the patient should be optimally referred to a center or specialist with a good experience of POTS. HUT

Table 13.2 The characteristic clinical presentation of POTS with associated symptoms

Cardiovascular symptoms	
Cardiovascular system	Main: *Orthostatic intolerance, orthostatic tachycardia, palpitations, dizziness, lightheadedness, (pre-) syncope, exercise intolerance.* Other frequent symptoms: Dyspnea, chest pain/discomfort, acrocyanosis, venous pooling, limb oedema
Non-cardiovascular symptoms (accompanying)	
General symptoms	General deconditioning, chronic fatigue, exhaustion, heat intolerance
Nervous system	Headache/migraine, mental clouding (brain fog), cognitive impairment, concentration problems, anxiety, tremulousness, sleeping disorders, light and sound sensitivity, blurred/tunnel vision, neuropathic pain (regional), involuntary movements
Musculoskeletal system	Muscle fatigue, weakness, muscle pain
Gastrointestinal system	Nausea, dysmotility, gastroparesis, constipation, diarrhea, abdominal pain, weight loss
Respiratory system	Hyperventilation, shortness of breath
Urogenital system	Bladder dysfunction, nycturia, polyuria
Skin	Petechiae, rashes, erythema, telangiectasia, diaphoresis, abnormal sudomotor regulation, pallor, flushing.

Adapted from: Fedorowski A. Postural orthostatic tachycardia syndrome: clinical presentation, aetiology and management. Journal of internal medicine. 2019;285(4):352–66

with a detailed noninvasive beat-to-beat hemodynamic monitoring is a crucial examination but usually requires both well-equipped laboratory and diagnostic skills to avoid over- and underdiagnosing. A panel of additional tests may be performed to explore the hemodynamic profile of patient, the possibility of coexisting inappropriate sinus tachycardia, to differentiate between the "hyperadrenergic" and "neuropathic" form, and to grade the symptoms.

13.2.2 Treatment

The management of POTS is usually focused on symptom alleviation [51, 52]. After the diagnosis has been established, patient should be thoroughly educated about nonpharmacological measures alleviating the symptoms, expected chronicity of symptoms, and available therapeutic options adequate to patient's status [30, 35, 48, 51–53] (Table 13.3). Here, the emphasis should be on patient's education, including avoidance of orthostatic intolerance triggers and better understanding of POTS pathophysiology. Exercise training may be very effective and has been shown to alleviate the symptoms of POTS-related deconditioning [54, 55]. If symptoms are pronounced, as evaluated by different score systems such as Orthostatic Hypotension Questionnaire (OHQ) [56], and functional class "pyramid" [2] focusing on complaints associated with orthostatic intolerance, or Karnofsky Performance Status [57] focusing on overall function limitation, the pharmacologic treatment should be considered. The most widely used drugs are presented in Table 13.3. However, it

Table 13.3 Different treatment options in postural orthostatic tachycardia syndrome. Of note: most of these treatment modalities may be applied in the treatment of orthostatic hypotension and recurrent vasovagal syncope

Therapy	Comments
Nonpharmacological treatment	
Education of patient: • Understanding of orthostatic intolerance and POTS pathophysiology • Avoidance of immobilization, prolonged recumbency, and physical deconditioning • Gradual rising from supine and sitting position, especially in the morning, after meals, and after urination/defecation • Small and frequent instead of large meals • Avoidance of prolonged standing, high ambient temperature, and high humidity • Physical counter-maneuvers (leg crossing, muscle tensing, squatting, etc.) during standing and prodromal symptoms [22, 59, 60]	This intervention is crucial and should be the fundamental of treatment strategy. It is rarely sufficient alone when pronounced symptoms are present. Patients and their families should understand the basics of orthostatic physiology and importance of nonpharmacological methods. Educational materials such as brochures and instruction films may be very helpful
Exercise training	There are different programs available. A regular, structured, and supervised exercise program featuring aerobic reconditioning is preferable. Initial training should avoid upright position. Mild to moderate intensity endurance training, progressing from semi-recumbent to upright position plus strength training is recommended. Rowing machines, recumbent bicycles, and swimming may be applied. Class IIA recommendation
Increased salt and fluid intake incl. peroral water bolus if needed	Volume expansion. A daily dietary intake of more than 10 g of sodium per day or salt tablets (e.g., 1 g TID) and a fluid intake of at least 2.5 L/day is recommended. This method is especially effective in "hypovolemic" subtype. Class IIB recommendation
Compression stockings/garments	Reduction of peripheral pooling in the lower limbs and splanchnic region. In general, Class 2 compression garments (>30 mmHg) are recommended. Especially when venous pooling is observed or suspected
Pharmacological treatments	
Heart rate controlling agents	
Beta-blockers propranolol, 10–40 mg TID bisoprolol, 2.5–5 mg BID metoprolol, 25–100 mg daily atenolol, 12.5–50 mg daily	Beta-blockers are especially recommended in "hyperadrenergic" subtype associated with sinus tachycardia >120 bpm on standing. Of note: beta-blockers may aggravate orthostatic intolerance in low-BP phenotype, asthma, and paroxysmal chest pain. Class IIB recommendation

Table 13.3 (continued)

Therapy	Comments
Ivabradine (2.5–7.5 mg BID)	This drug is effective when beta-blockers are not well tolerated. The evidence is based on small patient series
Verapamil (40–80 mg BID/TID)	This calcium channel blocker with negative chronotropic effect can be tested in "hyperadrenergic" type associated with higher BP, migraine, and chest pain. The evidence and clinical experience are very limited
Vasoactive and volume-expanding agents	
Clonidine (0.2–0.6 mg BID)	Centrally acting α2-adrenoreceptor agonist with overall sympatholytic effect. It is generally recommended for "hyperadrenergic" subtype and hypertensive tendency on standing. Class IIB recommendation according to current American guidelines
Midodrine (2.5–10 mg TID)	Direct α1-adrenoreceptor agonist. One of the few pharmacological agents positively tested in placebo-controlled studies for orthostatic hypotension. It may be effective in low-BP phenotype with pronounced orthostatic intolerance. Class IIB recommendation
Droxidopa (Northera, DOPS, 100–600 mg TID)	Peroral norepinephrine precursor. Drug is recommended in neurogenic OH and has been empirically used off-label in severe POTS. Not included in the current guidelines
Pyridostigmine (30–60 mg BID/TID)	Acetylcholinesterase inhibitor. It might be considered in POTS-phenotype associated with suspected autonomic neuropathy, gastrointestinal dysfunction, and nonspecific muscle weakness. Effect on BP is small. Class IIB recommendation
Fludrocortisone (0.1–0.2 mg daily)	Mineralocorticoid. Volume expander. Increases sodium reabsorption and enhances sensitivity of α-adrenoreceptors. May worsen supine hypertension and hypokalemia. It is recommended in low-BP phenotype. Class IIB recommendation
Ephedrine and pseudoephedrine (25/30–50/60 mg TID)	Direct and indirect α1-adrenoreceptor agonist. Efficacy is controversial
Desmopressin (0.1–0.4 mg BID)	Vasopressin analogue. Volume expander. Increases water reabsorption and reduces nycturia. Sparse evidence exists. Efficacy is uncertain
In-hospital acute 1–2 L physiological saline infusion (during consecutive 3–5 days)	In acute decompensated POTS, this method should be considered to alleviate the short-term symptoms. Class IIA recommendation.

BP blood pressure

Adapted from: Fedorowski A. Postural orthostatic tachycardia syndrome: clinical presentation, aetiology and management. Journal of internal medicine. 2019;285(4):352–66 should be kept in mind that large randomized trials are lacking [58], there are no Class I recommendations to date [28], and the only Class IIA recommendations are exercise training and acute saline infusion in decompensated POTS [28]. Among Class IIB recommendations are increased fluid and salt intake, midodrine, beta-blockers, fludrocortisone, pyridostigmine, clonidine, and alpha-methyldopa [28]. Consequently, the physician is often left alone with a decision which drug to test. Typically, clinicians test various drugs directed at controlling heart rate, increasing peripheral vasoconstriction, and increasing intravascular volume (Table 13.3). The overall effects of pharmacological therapy are modest, and the most symptomatic patients remain severely affected by the disease even if combination of different drugs is applied [28, 58].

13.3 Reflex Syncope

In accordance with the most recent guidelines from the European Society of Cardiology, syncope is defined as "*transient loss of consciousness (TLOC) due to cerebral hypoperfusion, characterized by a rapid onset, short duration, and spontaneous complete recovery*" [12]. The brain is critically dependent on stable perfusion, and if the cerebral blood flow is stopped for about 6 s or more, the likely outcome is complete loss of consciousness. Similarly, an SBP of 50–60 mmHg, meaning a BP of 30–45 mmHg at brain level in sitting or standing, will result in loss of consciousness [61, 62].

Whereas there are many alternative causes of TLOC, including epileptic seizures and traumatic TLOC, the mechanisms of syncope may be broadly divided into one of the three categories reflex syncope, OH, and primary cardiac syncope. This section will cover reflex syncope.

The broad term reflex syncope in turn involves the entities *vasovagal syncope*, *situational syncope*, and *carotid sinus syndrome* (the latter will be described in a separate section).

Vasovagal syncope, also known as *neurocardiogenic* syncope, is the most common mechanism of syncope [12]. In brief, vasovagal syncope is characterized by the following hallmarks:

- occurs during an upright posture or in conjunction with emotional stress, pain, or medical procedures;
- involves autonomic activation symptoms such as sweating, warmth, nausea, and pallor [63];
- is associated with hypotension and bradycardia in the final phase [63]; and
- after an episode of vasovagal syncope, the patient experiences fatigue [28].

If reflex syncope is triggered, or if there is an excessive BP decrease, during specific, well-defined physiologic situations, the syncope is classified as *situational syncope*. Situational syncope may be triggered by micturition, gastrointestinal stimulation (swallowing or defecation), coughing, sneezing, after exercise, or during other specific situations involving physiologic maneuvers such as laughing or playing a brass instrument [12].

Vasovagal syncope is extremely common. Studies have shown that by the age of 60, four out of ten women and three out of ten men will have experienced vasovagal syncope [64], even though most subjects may have had only one or a few episodes [28]. The first episode of vasovagal syncope usually occurs before the age of 40, with a median age of the first episode of 14 years [65]. In the elderly, vasovagal syncope may occur in conjunction with delayed OH in which the orthostatic BP decrease may trigger the vasovagal reflex, in turn resulting in complete syncope [4].

Vasovagal syncope usually occurs in otherwise healthy subjects and is not associated with any excess mortality. However, subjects with frequently occurring episodes suffer a significant loss of quality of life [28].

The physiology of vasovagal syncope is still not entirely clear. In general, vasovagal syncope is the result of the combination of bradycardia with subsequent reduction in cardiac output and vascular dilatation. The latter phenomenon is known as vasodepression and usually begins prior to the bradycardia [66]. The modified VASIS classification [67, 68] divides the response of the vasovagal syncope into a number of categories based on the involvement of bradycardia and vasodepression, respectively (Table 13.4).

Table 13.4 Modified classification of vasovagal syncope based on the heart rhythm behavior during loss of consciousness (modified from reference [68], Brignole et al.)

Type 1 Mixed	At the time of syncope, the ventricular rate either: • decreases to ≥40 bpm OR • decreases to <40 bpm for less than 10 s with or without asystole for 3 s AND • blood pressure decreases before the heart rate
Type 2 A	At the time of syncope, the ventricular rate: • decreases to <40 bpm for more than 10 s but without asystole for 3 s AND • blood pressure decreases before the heart rate
Type 2B	At the time of syncope: • asystole occurs for more than 3 s. AND • heart rate fall coincides with or precedes the blood pressure decrease
Type 3	At the time of syncope: • heart rate decreases no more than 10%, from its highest value
Exception 1: Chronotropic incompetence	No heart rate increase during orthostatic provocation (i.e., less than 10% increase from the supine position, meaning chronotropic incompetence)
Exception 2: Excessive heart rate increase	Excessive heart rate increase in the upright position prior to syncope

Diagnosis

The first step in the diagnostic process of reflex syncope is to confirm that the episode(s) of TLOC is caused by syncope (please see the definition at the beginning of this chapter), and not by potential differential causes such as epileptic seizures or psychogenic episodes. Sometimes, this step is quite simple, while in other situations, assessing the likely cause of TLOC may be rather challenging. If syncope turns out to be the likely cause of TLOC, the next step is to examine the specific underlying mechanism [12].

Vasovagal syncope could most often be diagnosed by careful history taking, searching for the clinical hallmarks of vasovagal syncope, described previously in this section. For example, vasovagal syncope is highly probable as the underlying diagnosis if the patient describes syncopal episodes that are precipitated by pain, fear, or standing and is associated with typical progressive prodromes of autonomic activation, such as pallor, sweating, and/or nausea. Similarly, if syncope is trigged by specific physiological situations, such as micturition, gastrointestinal stimulation, cough, sneeze, or postexercise, a diagnosis of situational syncope is highly likely [12]. It should be noted that fine and coarse myoclonic movements may be seen during episodes of vasovagal syncope. Thus, it is important that episodes of vasovagal syncope are not mistaken for epileptic seizures, solely on the basis of these myoclonic movements. After syncope, the patient usually regains consciousness after 1 or 2 min (often even quicker), but complete recovery of the patient may take longer. After an episode of vasovagal syncope, the patient often suffers from fatigue, which can last for hours [28].

Even though a careful history in most cases will be enough in order to adequately diagnose reflex syncope, some cases, especially if there is retrograde amnesia of the patient and/or absence of observers of the episode(s), may be more challenging. In case of uncertainness, a number of investigations may aid in the diagnosis of reflex syncope:

- *The active standing test*, during which the patient by him/herself adapts an upright position from supine under repeated BP measurements, can be easily performed during the patient examination. The patient should be standing for at least 3 min. While the active standing test seldom reproduces reflex syncope, it may reveal OH as a potential differential or additional diagnosis.
- *The head-up tilt table test* (HUT) involves the use of prolonged passive orthostatic stress to assess whether patients have the autonomic substrate for vasovagal syncope. The most common protocol of HUT is performed at 60–70° tilt including 20 min of passive orthostatic provocation followed by optional nitroglycerin provocation (400 μg spray sublingually) [69]. Ideally, beat-to-beat BP and electrocardiogram (ECG) are continuously monitored during the test using a noninvasive validated method [13].

During HUT, most patients with a history of probable vasovagal syncope develop pre-syncope or syncope that can be diagnosed as vasovagal syncope based on the

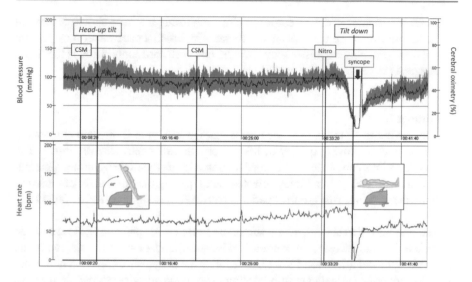

Fig. 13.3 Vasovagal syncope. Beat-to-beat blood pressure (mmHg) and cerebral oxygen saturation (%) in the upper panel with heart rate (bpm) depicted in red in the lower panel during head-up
tilt in a 68-year-old woman leading to an onset of vasovagal reflex and syncope after sublingual
nitroglycerine administration

reproduction of characteristic symptoms and the observation of physiological
changes typical for vasovagal syncope. In contrast, most subjects without a history
of syncope do not faint during HUT [70]. It is important to note that HUT, when
positive, merely suggests predisposition to vasovagal syncope and does not confirm
the cause [28]. That is, a positive HUT, including reproduction of symptoms along
with a characteristic circulatory pattern of vasovagal syncope, does suggest that a
vasovagal reflex is likely. However, a negative HUT does not exclude vasovagal
syncope as the underlying diagnosis [12]. A typical vasovagal reflex during HUT is
displayed in Fig. 13.3.

In adjunction to HUT, BP, heart rate, and ECG may be recorded during the
Valsalva maneuver. An excessive fall of BP during this test may occur in patients
with suspected situational syncope and may lead the thought of the physician to this
diagnosis.

- *Twenty-four hours ambulatory BP monitoring* may be used in order to detect
  diurnal changes in BP and whether symptoms suggestive of pre-syncope are
  indeed associated with episodes of low BP [12].
- *Prolonged electrocardiographic monitoring* may help the physician to correlate
  symptoms with arrhythmia. Whereas an episode with both sinus arrest and atrioventricular block during syncope is highly suggestive of vasovagal syncope with
  cardioinhibition, a syncope episode associated with normal sinus rhythm may
  still be due to reflex syncope with dominant vasodepression. A strategy involving
  the sequential use of carotid massage (described in detail under Sect. 13.3.2),

HUT, and prolonged electrocardiographic monitoring has been shown successful for identifying those patients aged >40 years in which a pacemaker may prevent syncope, probably because vasovagal syncope with cardioinhibition is the likely diagnosis in many of these cases [71].

Treatment

The benign nature of reflex syncope means that the treatment is directed at reducing symptoms and improving quality of life rather than influencing the prognosis. The treatment options can be divided into education and lifestyle interventions, pharmacological treatment, and, in highly selected cases, pacing therapy. Many of interventions are the same as in the group of patients with POTS, as summarized in Table 13.3.

The first line of treatment, which should be started in all patients without specific contraindications, involves reassurance, education, and general advice including adequate fluid and salt intake [28]. Of note, after the diagnosis of reflex syncope has been confirmed, most patients stop fainting even in the absence of specific therapy. Moreover, the number of episodes in the preceding year is highly predictive of the number of episodes in the coming year [72], meaning that in patient with no episodes in the recent year, a conservative approach is usually warranted.

The education of patients with vasovagal syncope includes recognizing the prodromal symptoms of autonomic activation and taking adequate countermeasures. This includes physical counter pressure maneuvers that can instantly increase BP, such as isometric activation of large muscle groups [60].

The pharmacological strategy that can be applied in reflex syncope involves medications that can increase or stabilize BP. Accounting for the high prevalence of comorbidities in elderly subjects, the first pharmacological intervention should be trying to reduce or optimize any agents that may decrease BP. Antihypertensive agents may be reduced or moved to the evening [2, 28, 73]. The next step in the pharmacological intervention strategy includes adding medications that may increase and stabilize BP. Midodrine is an alpha-agonist that increases vascular tone and has proved effective in small studies [12]. Fludrocortisone, another drug that may be used, works by increasing sodium retention, thereby increasing plasma volume and reducing the propensity to vasovagal reflex activation. This agent has shown a moderate effect on syncope in randomized trials [74]. Beta-blockers have been tried for preventing vasovagal reflex syncope, however, randomized trials have largely failed do demonstrate a positive effect [12].

The important therapy in vasovagal syncope is the implantation of a cardiac pacemaker, which may be effective in the case of dominant cardioinhibition [75]. Recent guidelines suggest that cardiac pacing should be considered in patients over 40 years, with spontaneous documented symptomatic asystolic pauses >3 s or asymptomatic pauses >6 s caused by sinus arrest and/or atrioventricular block [12]. Cardiac pacing may also be considered in patients over 40 years with frequently recurring unpredictable syncope, in whom HUT triggers asystole [12]. Of note, pacing therapy has shown to be more efficient, if HUT does not demonstrate a concurrent hypotensive susceptibility [76]. In case of asystole, the hypotensive susceptibility should be counteracted (for example, by decreasing antihypertensive agents) in order to potentially increase the efficacy of cardiac pacing [12].

13.3.1 Orthostatic Vasovagal Syncope

Vasovagal reflex syncope is commonly triggered during standing, especially during pronged standing in, for example, hot or crowded places, even though vasovagal reflex syncope may also occur in sitting in some situations. Vasovagal reflex syncope that occurs during these situations is usually referred to as *orthostatic vasovagal syncope* [12].

During the orthostatic vasovagal reflex, four phases can be observed, even though the time spent in each phase may vary [63]:

During *phase 1*, a change from supine to the upright position rapidly results in a shift of 0.5–1 L of blood volume from the thorax into vessels below the diaphragm, due to the gravitational forces. The reduction in central blood volume leads to a decrease in cardiac output, due to an incapacity of the heart rate to compensate for the fall in stroke volume. The compensation mechanisms during phase 1 involves baroreflex-mediated reflexes, which activate vasoconstriction in skeletal and splanchnic vascular beads, leading to increased systemic vascular resistance.

Phase 2 denotes the start of a circulatory instability and is characterized by a gradual fall in BP. Cardiac output falls in nearly all adult patients during this phase due to reduced central blood volume, whereas isolated vasodepression may occur in young patients.

Phase 3 involves the terminal hypotension, which results from a fall in cardiac output, with or without a fall in systemic vascular resistance. This phase involves a steep fall in BP and various involvement of bradycardia. This phase occurs at the same time as the development of the characteristic autonomic symptoms. Even though bradycardia is usually preceded by a fall in BP, some patients may develop asystole early during phase 3 with little or no warning, and these are the patients that, in selected cases, may benefit from pacing therapy [12, 75, 77].

The fourth and final phase involves the recovery of BP and heart rate after the patient has regained the supine position. During the supine position, there is an instant shift of blood from capacitance vessels below the diaphragm into the right atrium. This leads to rapid recovery of preload, stroke volume, and consequently cardiac output.

The phase 2 described above may vary in length and particularly in older subjects, and this phase may be of long duration. In some of these cases, this phase may correspond to delayed OH rather than vasovagal reflex activation. Delayed OH may in turn trigger the vasovagal reflex [4]. A typical such as is displayed in Fig. 13.2.

In the investigation of the physiology of Vasovagal syncope, a number of hormonal changes have been proposed as possible clues towards the mechanisms. Many studies converge on the role of epinephrine as a central hormone in Vasovagal syncope. The "epinephrine surge" hypothesis has been supported by several studies and stipulates that an early and greater rise in epinephrine contributes to the reflex as a trigger for vasovagal syncope; the higher the rise in epinephrine during initial phase of orthostatic provocation, the earlier vasovagal syncope occurs. Beside epinephrine, vasopressin and nitric oxide have been studied as possible contributors to vasovagal syncope [78, 79]. The diagnosis and treatment of orthostatic vasovagal syncope follows the treatment of vasovagal syncope in general and have been described in the previous section.

13.3.2 Carotid Sinus Syndrome

Reflex syncope that occurs with head rotation or pressure to the carotid sinus (such as shaving or with tight collars) suggests carotid sinus mediated reflex syncope. If pressure to the carotid sinus, such as during carotid sinus massage, leads to asystole for more than 3 s or a fall in BP of more than 50 mmHg from baseline, the condition is termed *carotid sinus hypersensitivity*. However, carotid sinus hypersensitivity is a common finding in older subjects without syncope, especially when there is coexisting CV disease. Accounting for this, the additional term *carotid sinus syndrome* is used only if there is carotid sinus hypersensitivity with simultaneous reproduction of syncope consistent with a reflex mechanism [12]. The prevalence of carotid sinus syndrome in subjects over 40 years was found to be 8.8% among 1800 patients that performed carotid sinus massage after the initial evaluation [80].

The etiology of carotid sinus syndrome is not completely understood. It is known that carotid sinus syndrome is a dysfunction of the autonomic nervous system, involving a pathological reflex resulting in cardioinhibition (via the vagus nerve) and vasodepression (due to withdrawal of sympathetic activity). This abnormal reflex is thought to result from disturbed carotid baroreceptor function and from degeneration of the medulla. There is an overlap between carotid sinus syndrome and vasovagal syncope, and these two entities may coexist in the same individual [81].

As described above, carotid sinus syndrome can be diagnosed by performing carotid sinus massage. Carotid sinus massage should be performed in patients aged over 40 years, with a history of syncope, unexplained falls, and presyncope and in whom the history, examination and CV, and neurological tests have not been diagnostic. The test must not be performed if the patient has had myocardial infarction, transient ischemic attack (TIA), or stroke in the preceding 3 months. In case of carotid bruits, ultrasound of the carotid artery should be performed, and carotid sinus massage should not be performed if there is a stenosis exceeding 70%.

Carotid sinus massage should be initially performed in the supine position, since most patients with carotid sinus hypersensitivity/syndrome show a positive response already in this position. In order to increase the chances of a diagnostic procedure, the patient should have surface electrocardiogram and BP monitoring (preferably beat to beat monitoring) during the whole procedure [13]. After excluding the contraindications described above, a distinct longitudinal massage should be applied

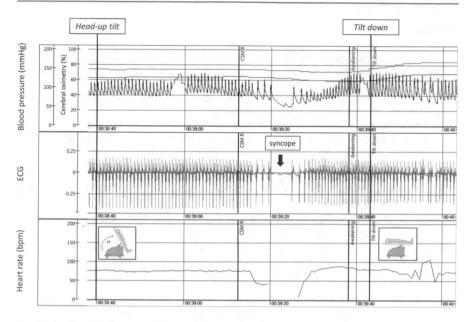

Fig. 13.4 Carotid sinus syndrome. Beat-to-beat blood pressure (mmHg) and cerebral oxygen saturation (%) in the upper panel with ECG and heart rate monitoring depicted in the middle and lower panels during tilt test in a 77-year-old man showing a typical response of carotid sinus syndrome (=sinus arrest of 6 s)

over the right carotid sinus for 5–10 s. The maximal pulsation of the carotid artery should be used in order to guide the site of the massage. It is important to note that pressure over the carotid sinus that is too weak or of too short duration will not produce a reliable response.

If there is no response (i.e., no asystole and/or fall in BP indicating carotid sinus hypersensitivity) on the right side, the same procedure that has been described is performed on the left side. Around one-third of subjects has carotid sinus hypersensitivity in standing position only, meaning that the procedure may have to be done also in upright position. This then does require a tilt table equipment [82].

Figure 13.4 shows a typical response of carotid sinus syndrome during head-up tilt testing.

Despite the lack of high-quality supporting data (i.e., randomized clinical trials), current guidelines recommend the consideration of a cardiac pacemaker in patients with carotid sinus syndrome with dominant cardioinhibition (i.e., asystole >3 s in combination with reproduction of syncope during provocation). In analogy to pacing for vasovagal syncope, any hypotensive susceptibility will decrease the effectiveness of such pacing, meaning that a low BP or OH should be targeted in order to increase the chance of a successful outcome of pacing [12, 83].

References

1. Freeman R, Wieling W, Axelrod FB, Benditt DG, Benarroch E, Biaggioni I, et al. Consensus statement on the definition of orthostatic hypotension, neurally mediated syncope and the postural tachycardia syndrome. Clin Auton Res. 2011;21(2):69–72.
2. Ricci F, De Caterina R, Fedorowski A. Orthostatic hypotension: epidemiology, prognosis, and treatment. J Am Coll Cardiol. 2015;66(7):848–60.
3. Torabi P, Ricci F, Hamrefors V, Sutton R, Fedorowski A. Classical and delayed orthostatic hypotension in patients with unexplained syncope and severe orthostatic intolerance. Front Cardiovasc Med. 2020;7:21.
4. Fedorowski A, van Wijnen VK, Wieling W. Delayed orthostatic hypotension and vasovagal syncope: a diagnostic dilemma. Clin Auton Res. 2017;27(4):289–91.
5. Streeten DH, Anderson GH Jr. Delayed orthostatic intolerance. Arch Intern Med. 1992;152(5):1066–72.
6. Gibbons CH, Freeman R. Delayed orthostatic hypotension: a frequent cause of orthostatic intolerance. Neurology. 2006;67(1):28–32.
7. van Wijnen VK, Finucane C, Harms MPM, Nolan H, Freeman RL, Westerhof BE, et al. Noninvasive beat-to-beat finger arterial pressure monitoring during orthostasis: a comprehensive review of normal and abnormal responses at different ages. J Intern Med. 2017;282(6):468–83.
8. Saedon NI, Pin Tan M, Frith J. The prevalence of orthostatic hypotension: a systematic review and meta-analysis. J Gerontol A Biol Sci Med Sci. 2020;75(1):117–22.
9. Gibbons CH, Freeman R. Clinical implications of delayed orthostatic hypotension: a 10-year follow-up study. Neurology. 2015;85(16):1362–7.
10. Dzau VJ, Antman EM, Black HR, Hayes DL, Manson JE, Plutzky J, et al. The cardiovascular disease continuum validated: clinical evidence of improved patient outcomes: part I: Pathophysiology and clinical trial evidence (risk factors through stable coronary artery disease). Circulation. 2006;114(25):2850–70.
11. Fedorowski A, Ricci F, Sutton R. Orthostatic hypotension and cardiovascular risk. Kardiol Pol. 2019;77(11):1020–7.
12. Brignole M, Moya A, de Lange FJ, Deharo JC, Elliott PM, Fanciulli A, et al. 2018 ESC Guidelines for the diagnosis and management of syncope. Eur Heart J. 2018;39(21):1883–948.
13. Brignole M, Moya A, de Lange FJ, Deharo JC, Elliott PM, Fanciulli A, et al. Practical instructions for the 2018 ESC Guidelines for the diagnosis and management of syncope. Eur Heart J. 2018;39(21):e43–80.
14. Tatasciore A, Zimarino M, Tommasi R, Renda G, Schillaci G, Parati G, et al. Increased short-term blood pressure variability is associated with early left ventricular systolic dysfunction in newly diagnosed untreated hypertensive patients. J Hypertens. 2013;31(8):1653–61.
15. Vallelonga F, Romagnolo A, Merola A, Sobrero G, Di Stefano C, Milazzo V, et al. Detection of orthostatic hypotension with ambulatory blood pressure monitoring in Parkinson's disease. Hypertens Res. 2019;42(10):1552–60.
16. Goldstein DS, Holmes C, Frank SM, Dendi R, Cannon RO 3rd, Sharabi Y, et al. Cardiac sympathetic dysautonomia in chronic orthostatic intolerance syndromes. Circulation. 2002;106(18):2358–65.
17. Boogers MJ, Borleffs CJ, Henneman MM, van Bommel RJ, van Ramshorst J, Boersma E, et al. Cardiac sympathetic denervation assessed with 123-iodine metaiodobenzylguanidine imaging predicts ventricular arrhythmias in implantable cardioverter-defibrillator patients. J Am Coll Cardiol. 2010;55(24):2769–77.
18. Shannon JR, Flattem NL, Jordan J, Jacob G, Black BK, Biaggioni I, et al. Orthostatic intolerance and tachycardia associated with norepinephrine-transporter deficiency. N Engl J Med. 2000;342(8):541–9.
19. Mills PB, Fung CK, Travlos A, Krassioukov A. Nonpharmacologic management of orthostatic hypotension: a systematic review. Arch Phys Med Rehabil. 2015;96(2):366–75.e6.

20. Pavelic A, Krbot Skoric M, Crnosija L, Habek M. Postprandial hypotension in neurological disorders: systematic review and meta-analysis. Clin Auton Res. 2017;27(4):263–71.
21. Jansen RW, Lipsitz LA. Postprandial hypotension: epidemiology, pathophysiology, and clinical management. Ann Intern Med. 1995;122(4):286–95.
22. Fedorowski A, Melander O. Syndromes of orthostatic intolerance: a hidden danger. J Intern Med. 2013;273(4):322–35.
23. Le Couteur DG, Fisher AA, Davis MW, McLean AJ. Postprandial systolic blood pressure responses of older people in residential care: association with risk of falling. Gerontology. 2003;49(4):260–4.
24. Schroeder C, Bush VE, Norcliffe LJ, Luft FC, Tank J, Jordan J, et al. Water drinking acutely improves orthostatic tolerance in healthy subjects. Circulation. 2002;106(22):2806–11.
25. Shibao C, Gamboa A, Diedrich A, Dossett C, Choi L, Farley G, et al. Acarbose, an alpha-glucosidase inhibitor, attenuates postprandial hypotension in autonomic failure. Hypertension. 2007;50(1):54–61.
26. Alam M, Smith G, Bleasdale-Barr K, Pavitt DV, Mathias CJ. Effects of the peptide release inhibitor, octreotide, on daytime hypotension and on nocturnal hypertension in primary autonomic failure. J Hypertens. 1995;13(12 Pt 2):1664–9.
27. Ong AC, Myint PK, Potter JF. Pharmacological treatment of postprandial reductions in blood pressure: a systematic review. J Am Geriatr Soc. 2014;62(4):649–61.
28. Sheldon RS, Grubb BP 2nd, Olshansky B, Shen WK, Calkins H, Brignole M, et al. 2015 heart rhythm society expert consensus statement on the diagnosis and treatment of postural tachycardia syndrome, inappropriate sinus tachycardia, and vasovagal syncope. Heart Rhythm. 2015;12(6):e41–63.
29. Fedorowski A. Postural orthostatic tachycardia syndrome: clinical presentation, aetiology and management. J Intern Med. 2019;285(4):352–66.
30. Arnold AC, Ng J, Raj SR. Postural tachycardia syndrome - diagnosis, physiology, and prognosis. Auton Neurosci. 2018;215:3–11.
31. Shaw BH, Stiles LE, Bourne K, Green EA, Shibao CA, Okamoto LE, et al. The face of postural tachycardia syndrome - insights from a large cross-sectional online community-based survey. J Intern Med. 2019;286(4):438–48.
32. Tanaka H, Monahan KD, Seals DR. Age-predicted maximal heart rate revisited. J Am Coll Cardiol. 2001;37(1):153–6.
33. Schondorf R, Low PA. Idiopathic postural orthostatic tachycardia syndrome: an attenuated form of acute pandysautonomia? Neurology. 1993;43(1):132–7.
34. Low PA, Opfer-Gehrking TL, Textor SC, Benarroch EE, Shen WK, Schondorf R, et al. Postural tachycardia syndrome (POTS). Neurology. 1995;45(4 Suppl 5):S19–25.
35. Stewart JM, Boris JR, Chelimsky G, Fischer PR, Fortunato JE, Grubb BP, et al. Pediatric disorders of orthostatic intolerance. Pediatrics. 2018;141(1):e20171673.
36. Thieben MJ, Sandroni P, Sletten DM, Benrud-Larson LM, Fealey RD, Vernino S, et al. Postural orthostatic tachycardia syndrome: the Mayo clinic experience. Mayo Clin Proc. 2007;82(3):308–13.
37. Hamrefors V, Spahic JM, Nilsson D, Senneby M, Sutton R, Melander O, et al. Syndromes of orthostatic intolerance and syncope in young adults. Open Heart. 2017;4(1):e000585.
38. Brinth LS, Pors K, Theibel AC, Mehlsen J. Orthostatic intolerance and postural tachycardia syndrome as suspected adverse effects of vaccination against human papilloma virus. Vaccine. 2015;33(22):2602–5.
39. Blitshteyn S, Brook J. Postural tachycardia syndrome (POTS) with anti-NMDA receptor antibodies after human papillomavirus vaccination. Immunol Res. 2017;65:282.
40. Watari M, Nakane S, Mukaino A, Nakajima M, Mori Y, Maeda Y, et al. Autoimmune postural orthostatic tachycardia syndrome. Ann Clin Transl Neurol. 2018;5(4):486–92.
41. Schofield JR, Hendrickson JE. Autoimmunity, autonomic neuropathy, and the HPV vaccination: a vulnerable subpopulation. Clin Pediatr (Phila). 2018;57(5):603–6.
42. Mathias CJ, Low DA, Iodice V, Owens AP, Kirbis M, Grahame R. Postural tachycardia syndrome-current experience and concepts. Nat Rev Neurol. 2012;8(1):22–34.

43. Garland EM, Celedonio JE, Raj SR. Postural tachycardia syndrome: beyond orthostatic intolerance. Curr Neurol Neurosci Rep. 2015;15(9):60.
44. McDonald C, Koshi S, Busner L, Kavi L, Newton JL. Postural tachycardia syndrome is associated with significant symptoms and functional impairment predominantly affecting young women: a UK perspective. BMJ Open. 2014;4(6):e004127.
45. Benarroch EE. Postural tachycardia syndrome: a heterogeneous and multifactorial disorder. Mayo Clin Proc. 2012;87(12):1214–25.
46. Boris JR, Bernadzikowski T. Demographics of a large paediatric Postural Orthostatic Tachycardia Syndrome Program. Cardiol Young. 2018;28(5):668–74.
47. Grubb BP. Postural tachycardia syndrome. Circulation. 2008;117(21):2814–7.
48. Zadourian A, Doherty TA, Swiatkiewicz I, Taub PR. Postural orthostatic tachycardia syndrome: prevalence, pathophysiology, and management. Drugs. 2018;78(10):983–94.
49. Shen WK, Sheldon RS, Benditt DG, Cohen MI, Forman DE, Goldberger ZD, et al. 2017 ACC/AHA/HRS Guideline for the evaluation and management of patients with syncope: executive summary: a report of the American College of Cardiology/American Heart Association Task Force on clinical practice guidelines and the Heart Rhythm Society. J Am Coll Cardiol. 2017;70(5):620–63.
50. Kavi L, Gammage MD, Grubb BP, Karabin BL. Postural tachycardia syndrome: multiple symptoms, but easily missed. Br J Gen Pract. 2012;62(599):286–7.
51. Miller AJ, Raj SR. Pharmacotherapy for postural tachycardia syndrome. Auton Neurosci. 2018;215:28–36.
52. Wells R, Spurrier AJ, Linz D, Gallagher C, Mahajan R, Sanders P, et al. Postural tachycardia syndrome: current perspectives. Vasc Health Risk Manag. 2018;14:1–11.
53. Goodman BP. Evaluation of postural tachycardia syndrome (POTS). Auton Neurosci. 2018;215:12–9.
54. Fu Q, Vangundy TB, Galbreath MM, Shibata S, Jain M, Hastings JL, et al. Cardiac origins of the postural orthostatic tachycardia syndrome. J Am Coll Cardiol. 2010;55(25):2858–68.
55. George SA, Bivens TB, Howden EJ, Saleem Y, Galbreath MM, Hendrickson D, et al. The international POTS registry: evaluating the efficacy of an exercise training intervention in a community setting. Heart Rhythm. 2016;13(4):943–50.
56. Kaufmann H, Malamut R, Norcliffe-Kaufmann L, Rosa K, Freeman R. The Orthostatic Hypotension Questionnaire (OHQ): validation of a novel symptom assessment scale. Clin Auton Res. 2012;22(2):79–90.
57. Peus D, Newcomb N, Hofer S. Appraisal of the Karnofsky Performance Status and proposal of a simple algorithmic system for its evaluation. BMC Med Inform Decis Mak. 2013;13:72.
58. Wells R, Elliott AD, Mahajan R, Page A, Iodice V, Sanders P, et al. Efficacy of therapies for postural tachycardia syndrome: a systematic review and meta-analysis. Mayo Clin Proc. 2018;93(8):1043–53.
59. Raj SR, Coffin ST. Medical therapy and physical maneuvers in the treatment of the vasovagal syncope and orthostatic hypotension. Prog Cardiovasc Dis. 2013;55(4):425–33.
60. Wieling W, van Dijk N, Thijs RD, de Lange FJ, Krediet CT, Halliwill JR. Physical countermeasures to increase orthostatic tolerance. J Intern Med. 2015;277(1):69–82.
61. Wieling W, Thijs RD, van Dijk N, Wilde AA, Benditt DG, van Dijk JG. Symptoms and signs of syncope: a review of the link between physiology and clinical clues. Brain. 2009;132(Pt 10):2630–42.
62. van Dijk JG, Thijs RD, van Zwet E, Tannemaat MR, van Niekerk J, Benditt DG, et al. The semiology of tilt-induced reflex syncope in relation to electroencephalographic changes. Brain. 2014;137(Pt 2):576–85.
63. Jardine DL, Wieling W, Brignole M, Lenders JWM, Sutton R, Stewart J. The pathophysiology of the vasovagal response. Heart Rhythm. 2018;15(6):921–9.
64. Ganzeboom KS, Mairuhu G, Reitsma JB, Linzer M, Wieling W, van Dijk N. Lifetime cumulative incidence of syncope in the general population: a study of 549 Dutch subjects aged 35-60 years. J Cardiovasc Electrophysiol. 2006;17(11):1172–6.

65. Sheldon RS, Sheldon AG, Connolly SJ, Morillo CA, Klingenheben T, Krahn AD, et al. Age of first faint in patients with vasovagal syncope. J Cardiovasc Electrophysiol. 2006;17(1):49–54.
66. Wieling W, Jardine DL, de Lange FJ, Brignole M, Nielsen HB, Stewart J, et al. Cardiac output and vasodilation in the vasovagal response: an analysis of the classic papers. Heart Rhythm. 2016;13(3):798–805.
67. Brignole M, Menozzi C, Del Rosso A, Costa S, Gaggioli G, Bottoni N, et al. New classification of haemodynamics of vasovagal syncope: beyond the VASIS classification. Analysis of the pre-syncopal phase of the tilt test without and with nitroglycerin challenge. Vasovagal Syncope International Study. Europace. 2000;2(1):66–76.
68. Brignole M, Tomaino M, Gargaro A. Vasovagal syncope with asystole: the role of cardiac pacing. Clin Auton Res. 2017;27(4):245–51.
69. Bartoletti A, Alboni P, Ammirati F, Brignole M, Del Rosso A, Foglia Manzillo G, et al. 'The Italian Protocol': a simplified head-up tilt testing potentiated with oral nitroglycerin to assess patients with unexplained syncope. Europace. 2000;2(4):339–42.
70. Sutton R, Brignole M. Twenty-eight years of research permit reinterpretation of tilt-testing: hypotensive susceptibility rather than diagnosis. Eur Heart J. 2014;35(33):2211–2.
71. Brignole M, Ammirati F, Arabia F, Quartieri F, Tomaino M, Ungar A, et al. Assessment of a standardized algorithm for cardiac pacing in older patients affected by severe unpredictable reflex syncopes. Eur Heart J. 2015;36(24):1529–35.
72. Pournazari P, Sahota I, Sheldon R. High remission rates in vasovagal syncope: systematic review and meta-analysis of observational and randomized studies. JACC Clin Electrophysiol. 2017;3(4):384–92.
73. Solari D, Tesi F, Unterhuber M, Gaggioli G, Ungar A, Tomaino M, et al. Stop vasodepressor drugs in reflex syncope: a randomised controlled trial. Heart. 2017;103(6):449–55.
74. Sheldon R, Raj SR, Rose MS, Morillo CA, Krahn AD, Medina E, et al. Fludrocortisone for the prevention of vasovagal syncope: a randomized, placebo-controlled trial. J Am Coll Cardiol. 2016;68(1):1–9.
75. Sutton R, de Jong JSY, Stewart JM, Fedorowski A, de Lange FJ, et al. Heart Rhythm. 2020;17(5 Pt A):821–8.
76. Brignole M, Donateo P, Tomaino M, Massa R, Iori M, Beiras X, et al. Benefit of pacemaker therapy in patients with presumed neurally mediated syncope and documented asystole is greater when tilt test is negative: an analysis from the third International Study on Syncope of Uncertain Etiology (ISSUE-3). Circ Arrhythm Electrophysiol. 2014;7(1):10–6.
77. Yasa E, Ricci F, Holm H, Persson T, Melander O, Sutton R, et al. Pacing therapy in the management of unexplained syncope: a tertiary care centre prospective study. Open Heart. 2019;6(1):e001015.
78. Fedorowski A, Sutton R. Understanding vasovagal syncope akin to the philosopher's stone? J Cardiovasc Electrophysiol. 2019;30(3):297–8.
79. Torabi P, Ricci F, Hamrefors V, Melander O, Sutton R, Benditt DG, et al. Impact of cardiovascular neurohormones on onset of vasovagal syncope induced by head-up tilt. J Am Heart Assoc. 2019;8(12):e012559.
80. Solari D, Maggi R, Oddone D, Solano A, Croci F, Donateo P, et al. Clinical context and outcome of carotid sinus syndrome diagnosed by means of the 'method of symptoms'. Europace. 2014;16(6):928–34.
81. Sutton R. Carotid sinus syndrome: progress in understanding and management. Glob Cardiol Sci Pract. 2014;2014(2):1–8.
82. Parry SW, Reeve P, Lawson J, Shaw FE, Davison J, Norton M, et al. The Newcastle protocols 2008: an update on head-up tilt table testing and the management of vasovagal syncope and related disorders. Heart. 2009;95(5):416–20.
83. Yasa E, Ricci F, Holm H, Persson T, Melander O, Sutton R, et al. Cardiovascular autonomic dysfunction is the most common cause of syncope in paced patients. Front Cardiovasc Med. 2019;6(154):154.

Index

Printed in the United States
by Baker & Taylor Publisher Services